A PLUME BOOK

GRATITUDE AND TRUST

PAUL WILLIAMS is an Oscar-, Grammy-, and Golden Globe–winning Hall of Fame songwriter ("Rainbow Connection," "Evergreen," and "We've Only Just Begun") and president of the American Society of Composers, Authors and Publishers (ASCAP). He is a major public force in the recovery movement, a graduate of UCLA's Drug and Alcohol Counseling Certification Program and has served as a member of the National Council on Alcoholism and Drug Dependence Board of Directors. He was a founding board member and counselor for the Musicians Assistance Program (MAP), now the treatment wing of MusiCares. He has been a passionate public advocate for the recovery movement for the past twenty-four years.

TRACEY JACKSON wrote the films *Confessions of a Shopaholic*, *The Guru*, and *The Other End of the Line*, among others. She has also written twelve TV pilots and created the series *Babes* for Fox TV. Tracey wrote, directed, and starred in the controversial documentary *Lucky Ducks*, which can presently be seen on Amazon, Journeyman Docs, and pay-per-view. Her first book, *Between a Rock and a Hot Place: Why Fifty is Not the New Thirty*, came out in 2011 and was optioned for a TV movie by Lifetime.

Praise for *Gratitude and Trust*

"This amazing book is about a revolutionary concept—recovery for the non-addict, for those who have longed for what their recovering friends have: a spiritual path, healthy company, and a little light to see by. Paul Williams and Tracey Jackson have great insight into our shared problems, solutions, humanity, craziness, and dreams. Plus, they will make you laugh, and give you hope, that recovery—starting over—is for everyone who has imagined a life of immediacy, honesty, and joy." —Anne Lamott

"What a great gift—Christmas, Hanukkah, holidays—to give *Gratitude and Trust*." —Oprah Winfrey, *Super Soul Sunday*

"Personal and powerful . . . An amazing book." —Kathie Lee Gifford

ALSO BY TRACEY JACKSON

Between a Rock and a Hot Place

Gratitude & Trust

SIX AFFIRMATIONS THAT WILL
CHANGE YOUR LIFE

Paul Williams &
Tracey Jackson

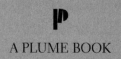

A PLUME BOOK

PLUME
An imprint of Penguin Random House LLC
375 Hudson Street
New York, New York 10014
penguin.com

First published in the United States of America by Blue Rider Press,
an imprint of Penguin Random House LLC, 2014
First Plume Printing 2015

THE LIBRARY OF CONGRESS HAS CATALOGED THE BLUE RIDER PRESS EDITION
AS FOLLOWS:

Williams, Paul, date.
Gratitude and trust : six affirmations that will change your life /
Paul Williams and Tracey Jackson.
p.   cm.
ISBN 978-0-399-16719-5 (hc.)
ISBN 978-0-14-751796-8 (pbk.)
1. Change (Psychology).   2. Compulsive behavior.   3. Self-control.
4. Affirmations.   5. Twelve-step programs.   I. Jackson, Tracey.
II. Title.
BF637.C4W553   2014   2014022844
158.1—dc23

Printed in the United States of America
10 9 8 7 6 5 4 3 2 1

Original hardcover design by Amanda Dewey

For Blink—This one's for you

Blake Snyder, October 3, 1957–August 4, 2009

For Jerry H.—Who led me to the light

Jerry M. Hunter, August 27, 1932–August 17, 2004

CONTENTS

Gratitude
& Trust

Thus I believe the greatest positive event of the twentieth century occurred in Akron, Ohio, on June 10, 1935, when Bill W. and Dr. Bob convened the first AA meeting. It was not only the beginning of the self-help movement and the beginning of the integration of science and spirituality at a grass-roots level, but also the beginning of the community movement.

That is the other reason why I think of addiction as the sacred disease. When my AA friends and I get together, we often come to conclude that, very probably, God deliberately created the disorder of alcoholism in order to create alcoholics, in order that these alcoholics might create AA, and thereby spearhead the community movement which is going to be the salvation not only of alcoholics and addicts but of us all.

—M. SCOTT PECK,

Further Along the Road Less Traveled:
The Unending Journey Toward Spiritual Growth

INTRODUCTION

We all visualize a fairy-tale version of what our lives will ultimately look like or are right now. Maybe it starts out with the little boy who wants to be a superhero and save people from burning buildings, or it's the little girl who dreams of being a ballerina in pretty pink slippers and being swept around the stage by Prince Charming. But while some childhood fantasies are sometimes realized, they often get left behind for more reachable, basic goals. Most people settle for a job—hopefully a fulfilling one—that brings in a livable wage. It doesn't always have to be heroic or Forbes 400 material, just something to pay the bills. Most healthy people long for a nurturing relationship with a partner and maybe a few children to love and raise into adulthood—preferably children who will love them back and cause as little turbulence as possible. We all seek healthy, sustaining friendships; fit bodies; positive attitudes; clean lives; and unpolluted souls. We set goals and cross our fingers that we can achieve them. Or at least we want to set goals and achieve them. But mostly we want to live lives unburdened by anger, resentment, and bad habits.

But the truth is, life seldom turns out the way we imagined it would through the eyes of childhood innocence. More often than not, hard knocks and cold realities change the Disney version of a life into one we barely recognize. Family members are damaged and narcissistic, jobs don't always turn out the way we want, and our own demons prevent us from capturing the flag and running with it. We give up on diets, friendships, love affairs, and our higher goals. We make poor choices that are steeped in our fears and not our abilities. We see the truth in negative feedback and don't rely on our own talents or the help of a higher power. We then find ourselves staring in the mirror and not liking who we see. But we are either too frightened or shackled by a lifetime of poor choices that have become habits to know how to change it. We live lives that are limited by our own actions. We may not be lying in a gutter with a needle hanging out of our arm, but the path we are on is not the one we dreamt about, chose, or even want to stay on.

But how do we change paths midlife? How do we turn it all around midstream? In fact, how do we even identify what the "it" is that needs to change? Far too often we have that niggling feeling something is amiss, but what we are not sure about is what.

Life is never going to be perfect; it has too many moving parts. And the adolescent dreams of a child may have no real place in the chaos of adulthood. Yet, a happy, centered, purposeful, healthy, constructive, spiritual (if we so desire), fear-free life is attainable. A life where we set our goals and continuously strive to reach them. An existence where we take responsibility for our mistakes and turn them into lessons and not harbors of shame. A place where we understand that the world is not going to change just because we whine and scream and try to pound it into submission, but rather that the only part we have control over changing is ourselves, be it our actions or our attitude.

We're not promising to turn you into a superhero, but if you follow the path we set out for you in this book, we can promise that you will become productive, responsible, content, trusting, and grateful. With just six simple affirmations, six easy little tools, you will be on the road to faith and higher purpose that opens doors and windows you thought were forever locked. You'll learn to seek out healthy over destructive, nurture happy over sad, choose trust over fear. You'll replace debilitating relationships with life-enhancing ones. Or if they can't be replaced, you'll learn how to deal with them so they no longer suck the life out of you and cause you pain. And as you continue on this path, you'll finally be living the life you imagined for yourself.

By now you are likely saying, "Yeah, right. I've heard that one before." Or perhaps you might be muttering, "How can you do all that with just six 'easy' tools?"

Six it is. As for easy, nothing worth attaining is as easy as *abracadabra*. But good things *can* happen just because you want them to, and it starts with these tools. If you use the affirmations as we've laid them out, go back to them daily, keep them at the forefront of your consciousness, work hard to stay on the path, and persevere even when you want to give up and give in to your old habits and behaviors, we assure you that you will see results.

How do we know this to be true? Because these affirmations stem from the mother ship, aka the Oxford Group, which inspired the most successful recovery program to ever come along. So while we wrote each of these affirmations, they are concepts that have existed in various forms for ages. If you attempt to trace their beginnings, you'll find yourself traveling through the histories of some remarkable groups, organizations, and religions. You'll find teachings that support our thinking in Buddhism, Hinduism, Judeo-Christian main-stage rituals, and New Age/New Thought alterations and add-ons. You'll be led to the philosophy of William James and Ralph Waldo Emerson.

Our Six Affirmations are the children of the Four Absolutes and the Six Tenets of the Oxford Group and beyond. Or stepchildren, if you will. These absolutes are honesty, purity, unselfishness, and love. They are the basis for much of unadulterated religion, and over the decades they have gone on to help millions find their way out of the dark, tormented tunnel of addiction. But as M. Scott Peck says, they are the "salvation not only of alcoholics and addicts, but of us all."

PAL

Variations of these affirmations, many more religious in tone than ours, have worked for millions of people in different forms. And they have worked for Tracey and for me exactly as they are written here. If they hadn't, there would be no book. Our goal in writing the affirmations was simple, but achieving it has taken much more time, effort, and discipline than any of the songs I've written for over forty years. Rhyming is easier. But, we believed we'd found a way to share the gift of recovery in a new, easy-to-understand language. The affirmations work. We've used them all.

Honesty, Purity, Unselfishness, and Love

These four little words are the touchstone for a path to healing. Seems pretty simple when you see it spelled out like that, right?

It all starts with **honesty**. If you're not honest with yourself, how can you be truly honest with anyone else? We spend a lot of energy fooling ourselves, covering for ourselves, and projecting an image that is in opposition of what's actually going on. There is such an emphasis on perfection in our society that we are all terrified of not meeting the standards that we either self-imposed or assume the world is expecting of us. Changing that begins with honesty: being honest about who you are, where you are, what you feel, what you want, and where you might have dropped the ball. Honesty is not only the best policy, it's the starting line of getting through the race of life as smoothly as possible.

Purity in many ways is the cousin of honesty. Once you have decided to embrace honesty and let that be the controlling dynamic of your life, you must be pure to that concept. The definition of purity is cleanliness, transparency. So by following the path of purity, you keep your house clean and your personal life clean. You maintain transparency about your misdeeds and mistakes because when you're being transparent, you're being honest. And when we're honest, we have nothing to hide from ourselves and others. Addicts of all sorts spend their lives covering their tracks. But any of us who merely have dents in our character—which we all do—spend a lot of our lives trying to mask them, hide from them, numb them, and beat them into oblivion. Think about how much more time you will have to do the things you want and be the person you want when you are not constantly running from your reality trying to cover up the things you don't want to be or do.

Unselfishness is not just "Let's all be Mother Teresa and give up our lives for others." That is unrealistic and extreme. Being unselfish is not just putting others before ourselves. It's being generous, kind, and considerate. It's treating others the way you yourself want to be treated. Or as Franklin Roosevelt said: "Confidence thrives on honesty, on honor, on the sacredness of obligations, on faithful protection and on unselfish performance. Without them it cannot live."

Also, as they say in recovery, "You get to keep the gift by giving it away." By being unselfish you don't simply make others feel good, but in the act of doing so, you build your own confidence. And when we come from a place of confidence, our decisions tend to be healthier and more sensible. We are not operating from fear and weakness but rather from strength. Our heads are clear and our hearts are full. Unselfishness is the birthplace of gratitude.

As for **Love**—"what the world needs now," right?—it's been a theme of life since Adam and Eve. No word or feeling has inspired so much art, music, literature, film, and dreams. *Love* is one of those words that gets tossed around in songs and poems and can often be labeled as sappy and sentimental. But it is what we all yearn for: to love and be loved. To love ourselves, to be loved and respected by others. Familial love, the love of friends, the love we feel for our pets. It is the ultimate connection. In its purest form, it is untethered by conditions, needs, or stipulations. It just *is*. That can be hard to find and easy to lose.

We long to give it freely, receive it elegantly. It comforts and protects. It erases competition, anger, hurt, and fear. It's so powerful that people are frightened of it. They often run from it. What if they accept love and it is removed? That is an example of dealing from fear and not confidence.

And by the way, how did "us all" get left out of that banquet of riches that M. Scott Peck refers to? A banquet of riches that has allowed millions of people to transform their lives from unbearable and destitute to vibrant and beautiful. Even though the recovery movement has migrated into other forms, such as eating, gambling, and sex addiction, it has never been offered to those of us who are not suffering from life-threatening behavior, just life-*limiting* behavior.

"Us all." That is who we have written this book for. That large group of people who have been left out of one of the greatest, longest-lasting, most proven roads to self-improvement of all. Because people are unhappy as hell and willing to do just about anything to take a stab at fixing it. And with this book, we plan on showing you how to do just that.*

PAUL
....

When Tracey came to me with the idea that there might be a way to share the process of recovery in an entirely new voice, I was excited. For years I've experienced the frustration of

---

*We are in no way underplaying, or minimizing, the destructive, severe, and sometimes life-threatening effects of the disease of alcoholism. Nor are we in any way comparing the nonalcoholic segment of the population who will be reading this book with those who are suffering from addiction.

friends dealing with life-limiting habits and wishing there
was a practice that would assist them in changing direction
and living a richer and more meaningful life.

The new life I've been given asks only that I be willing
to share the gift with others who suffer. This book offered
a wonderful way to do just that. The tradition of love and
service is but one promise I've made and will never break.

TRACEY

One of the most commonly heard phrases in "the rooms" is
"It's too bad the rest of the world doesn't have a program of
recovery." And those who are not part of the program but have
been exposed to it by either attending an open meeting with a
friend or family member, going to a sober birthday party, or
hearing secondhand of the methods and steps used to gain
sobriety often utter, "I wish I had something like that in
my life."

PAUL'S PATH

My name is Paul and I'm an alcoholic and an addict. Which is a little like saying you're from New York, New York.

You know you're an alcoholic when you misplace a decade. I misplaced the eighties. I had a brief affair with cocaine—an expensive little chemistry experiment that lasted almost twenty-five years. There were many years when someone else was using my body.

There is very little "Hemingway blood and guts" in my drunkalogue. I never emerged from a blackout with a Russian arms dealer. I never came to in a sleazy Parisian hotel with Norman Mailer and a couple of hookers. No, I'd come out of a blackout in the boys' department of Sears trying on sweaters; enveloped by suffocating yarn in the shape of a deformed reindeer. Alcoholic terrors: One size fits all.

I was raised in a home where alcohol was the reward for a hard day's work. My six-foot-plus father was a construction worker who fol-

lowed jobs from town to town. I attended nine schools by the time I was
in the eighth grade. Small for my age, I'd been given male hormone
shots to make me grow. The hormones had the opposite effect, causing
my bones to stop growing yet hurling me into puberty by the age of ten.
They quit the shots but the damage had been done. I suddenly found
myself more interested in the contents of my mother's friends' blouses
than what was inside my toy chest.

My father drank excessively and it eventually killed him. I was thirteen when he died in an alcohol-related car wreck. Due to the financial
difficulties my mother was experiencing, I was forced to move in with
an aunt who lived a thousand miles away. Thus, I basically lost my father and mother at the same time. A one-way ticket to isolation and the
fear of not belonging to anyone, anywhere, a situation that would plague
me for years to come.

Attending high school in Long Beach, California, I was an oddity.
Measuring in at only four feet six inches tall, the effects of early puberty
had disappeared and I was a teenager trapped in a child's body. I was in
my twenties before my body clock delivered me into adulthood.

The sense of belonging, fitting in, and being socially comfortable
came with the confidence alcohol *could* provide. I started drinking in
my teens. Although I don't know exactly when I crossed the line from
use to abuse to addiction, I can tell you that at the peak of my disease,
I began each day with a drink. Excessive? I didn't think so. I thought
everyone started their day with a glass of vodka in the shower.

Another form of comfort came with being an actor: Playing other
people was easier than being me. In my early twenties, still looking like
a little boy, I could be seen playing a thirteen-year-old—almost convinc-
ingly—in the dark comedy *The Loved One*. I looked like a kid until you
put me next to a real kid. Then I looked like a kid with a hangover. I'd

asked the universe to make me an actor. A star. I felt like Montgomery Clift or James Dean. I looked like Hayley Mills. The universe said no. *No*, I was to discover, is often a gift.

I had a small part in *The Chase* with Marlon Brando, and during the endless hours one sits on a set I began to doodle with a borrowed guitar. I can be seen in the film singing the first little ditty that I created. To soothe my troubled and saddened heart, I began to write songs for my own amusement. Songwriting changed everything. Signed by A&M Records, I began writing for many of the most successful artists of the time as well as the living legends of music. My songs were recorded by everyone from Elvis to Sinatra, Ella Fitzgerald to Miss Piggy. My walls started filling up with plaques and the shelves with awards. I was nominated for six Oscars, winning in 1977 for "Evergreen (Love Theme from *A Star Is Born*)," which I cowrote with Barbra Streisand. I had hits with Three Dog Night, the Carpenters, Helen Reddy, and Kermit the Frog. I won a Grammy for *The Muppet Movie* and the "Rainbow Connection."

The writing success led to recording my own songs and performing live before thousands, touring, television appearances, and more movies. I appeared on *The Tonight Show Starring Johnny Carson* forty-eight times. I remember six. I'd gone from feeling *different* to feeling *special*. Feeling *different* is difficult. Feeling *special* is addictive. I was suddenly elbow to elbow with the people I'd admired since childhood. I went from the odd outsider to the ultimate insider. A full-fledged member of the world's most desired club. I was a star. Yet my drinking increased. *How did I get here?* I'd wonder. *Do I really belong?*

I had an Oscar on my piano and a star on Hollywood Boulevard. It still wasn't enough. There was still a dark place deep inside my being where I continued to feel like the outcast.

Alcoholism is a progressive disease, and it wasn't long before my dependence led me to a place where leaving the house to work or perform was almost impossible. Isolation is often a characteristic of the sickness. It was only a matter of time before I'd traded sitting on Johnny's couch for hiding in my bedroom. Three a.m. and I'm loaded on cocaine, peeking out the venetian blinds, looking for the "tree police."

In 1986 I left my wife and children for a twenty-two-year-old psych major. A year and half into the relationship she informed me I was an alcoholic and an addict and that she loved me too much to watch me die. If I continued on this road she would leave me.

The idea of being alone was too much to even consider. A true codependent, I was afraid I'd vanish without her. Consumed by my addiction, I wasn't really capable of having a meaningful relationship. But I needed her. Like the life vest under the passenger seat on an airplane, she was my last hope for connecting to real life.

My drinking and using had progressed to the point where even simple conversation was difficult. Endless trips to the bathroom to have a secret hit of cocaine made my addiction pretty obvious. Erratic, slurred speech and jumping from one grandiose comment to another added to the image of a lost soul. And not a very nice one.

I drank around the clock and slept little, and when I did awaken, it was with a two-gram bottle of cocaine grasped tightly in my fist. I needed my medicine and I needed my lover at my side. The romanticized relationship was woven into my idea of a successful life. When she brought up my addiction and threatened to leave, I announced that I'd been thinking about getting help. "Somebody's whispering, honey.

I want to put this behind me." I didn't want any such thing. But I couldn't lose her.

In order to keep her at my side, I made a quick trip to a facility famous for aversion therapy. After being given an injection that makes you extremely ill, you're forced to drink huge amounts of liquor. All kinds. The thinking is that while you heave and heave to expel the offending liquor, you'll associate the sickness with the booze. The next day you're given an injection of Sodium Pentothal, or truth serum, and while under the influence you're asked if you want another drink. If you answer "Yes," you return the next day for additional heaving. After going through a few rounds of this, the counselors confessed they were worried about me. When I asked why, they told me I was the only patient who was always early for the Sodium Pentothal.

I kept drinking. She left. My drug and alcohol use increased. A year later, leaving a hotel room in Oklahoma City where I was booked to perform, I experienced a complete psychotic meltdown. After several days and nights without sleep, and with large quantities of cocaine and vodka in my bloodstream, I was literally out of my mind. Invisible monsters were shoving me down the stairs, twisting my ears, and biting me on the neck. I had finally lost it. I had hit the proverbial bottom. Or so I thought.

The promoter of the concert was horrified. The gig I'd come to play was postponed until the next day.

Taking illicit drugs and drinking were the only things I could do to fill the void in my chest and pacify the cravings. I'd become so dependent on the substances that I lived in a constant state of hunger for more. The high that had come with the early usage was gone forever.

I returned to Los Angeles to an empty house, where I continued to drink for a few weeks. Then, inexplicably, while I was blacked out, I called a doctor and asked him to find a place for me to be admitted. I needed rehab. I couldn't do it anymore. I was going to die.

And so my journey toward recovery began. I've been sober since March 15, 1990. The life I have today is beyond anything I could have imagined in the midst of my disease. I enjoy a new freedom and a new happiness.

The path I took to get here is the oldest and best hope for any alcoholic or addict who seeks help. The new life I've been given asks only that I share the gift with others who suffer, and it's a promise I've made and will never break. Because we get to keep the gift by giving it away. Nowhere in the writing of this book will that or any other recovery tradition be ignored.

For the last twenty-two years I have traveled the world, happy to share my experience, strength, and hope amongst my peers and often at a public level when my appearance would benefit our cause. My message is a simple one: There is hope for the hopeless. My warts-and-all story is meant to illustrate that no segment of society is immune to the devastating effects of addiction. Although the media devotes endless ink and camera time to the antics of the rich and famous, there is little difference between the rock star shooting heroin and the bored Indiana housewife drinking Listerine. (FYI, it is 28 percent alcohol.) Both are attempts to deal with pain, fear, or boredom by self-medicating with highly addictive substances. And under the influence of alcohol and other drugs, our impulse controls are often muted and our behavior becomes socially unacceptable. Atrocious. But, like the many divorces that are often the end result of untreated addiction, it's the celebrities who are offered to the public court of opinion.

I'm an advocate of recovery and am still as enthusiastic about the way of life today as I was in those first few sober days. How I found my way out of the darkness and into the light wasn't something I instigated or ever considered necessary, but still I woke up instead of coming to. A new life was waiting. And while *abstinence* had been my only goal, *sobriety* has offered more than I could have imagined. Medically detoxed and drug-free, I made a sober choice to accept the gift I was being given. The success I had known through my music had given me a one-step-removed connection to the rest of the world. It was an isolated perch that may have appeared to be enviable but in truth was a very lonely place to live. Recovery gave me a worldwide family and a simple guide to living life on life's terms. There are angels of change who played important roles in my recovery, and this book is a chance to offer the same sweet healing gift to you.

—Paul Williams

TRACEY'S PATH

I'm Tracey and I'm not an alcoholic. While I never turned to alcohol or drugs to self-soothe, I did plenty of other things. Men, cigarettes, overspending, and catastrophic thinking took the place of vodka and cocaine for several decades in my life.

It's not because of some overwhelmingly impressive personal strength that I was able to literally walk away from endless lines of coke sliced in front of me, hand back Quaaludes slipped to me at a dinner, or even refuse Hunter S. Thompson's pleas to take a hit off his hash pipe. I just wasn't interested. I was actually scared. I am one of the few people who believed the film *Reefer Madness*. You know when they make those films they say, "If we can prevent one person from turning to drugs, if after seeing this film one person says no to grass, LSD, shrooms (okay they probably didn't say *shrooms*, but I don't want to come off as a total simp), that one person will make this film a success and we will have done our job." Okay, producers of *Reefer Madness*, you did it! Home run! I totally bought into marijuana being a one-way ticket to heroin addiction. I walked out of that film and Just Said No to so many drugs, I could have been Nancy Reagan's poster girl.

Though I said yes to many men whose names I now can't remember and at the time my phone number was the first thing they forgot.

I would like to say to the producers of *Reefer Madness*: While you were making lifesaving films, you should have done one called *Just Because He Wants to Sleep with You Doesn't Mean He Will Love You a Lot and Make Up for the Fact That Your Father Doesn't*.

But back to my inner Nancy Reagan. I'm also a control freak. I suffer from panic disorder and OCD, which manifests itself in my obsession with everything having to be in total order, all the time, so the idea of losing control was and is far more frightening to me than the concept of pain-numbing drugs was appealing. Even though I had enough pain that required numbing, I chose a different brand of Band-Aid to cover it.

While my career was glamorous and steady, it was not as high-voltage as Paul's. My childhood was isolated and lonely in many of the same ways his was, though. I too felt like I never belonged. Tolstoy says, "Happy families are all alike; but every unhappy family is unhappy in its own way." I'm not sure a comedy writer should be arguing with Tolstoy, but I disagree, Leo, at least when it comes to children. I think most children who are unhappy are unhappy for many of the same reasons, and thus often in the same way.

Like 50 percent of parents, mine split up. They did so when I was four. I don't think divorce undermines a child's security in the absolute, but it certainly calls much of it into question. My father had a bit of the magician in him. He had the ability to vanish, then reappear with amazing regularity. He wasn't a deadbeat dad per se; he was just indifferent or often angry with me for no apparent reason. Years would pass when I would not see him at all. He would fight with my mother or create some unspoken displeasure with me that sent him away for two or more years at a time. I never really understood why, which resulted in a character trait that would take me four decades to shake: thinking everything that ever went wrong was my fault.

We lived in a small town, so I would occasionally run into my father when we were in an off period. The episode that stands out most is being seven and seeing him at the supermarket. He pushed his cart past me without saying a word. That alone might set up a lifelong pattern of reaching out to the wrong men to love you: righting the wrongs of your past by choosing wrongs in your present. Also, I was not popular in school. I grew up very fast in order to be my mother's friend, and kids don't want to hang out with grown-ups, especially grown-ups who happen to be their age.

While I find it annoying to hear successful grown-ups whine about their childhoods and blame all their problems on their parents, I think many people carry pain from when they were young and it influences most if not all of their maladaptive patterned behavior, which they are doomed to repeat unless they fix it. So not feeling like I belonged was something that fueled my life in the same way it fueled Paul's.

I suppose this is the place to tell you that the music I mainly listened to in my early teens was Paul's. He was writing what I was feeling, even if I didn't really know it. I just knew it made me feel not so alone.

I too turned to drama: being someone else was easier for me. Like Paul's, my acting career did not pan out, but in trying to express myself in some way, I turned to writing. It was one of the big Aha! moments of my life. I sat down and was suddenly able to write down the deeper feelings I was never able to express. It was the first time in my life an entire day could pass without my bothering to look at the clock because I was so immersed in what I was doing. I had the ability to make sense of certain events in my life by turning them into comedies.

Comedy was what really saved me. Funny means you can make jokes at your own expense and others'. It means you see the world through a scrim that makes even raw and painful situations amusing. It puts distance between you and your pain. But the drawback to this is it can also put off the act of dealing with the pain. When you spend a lot of time making light of things that are heavy, it ultimately means you don't deal with them until you have some sort of crisis. Most funny people are not happy people. The trick is getting healthy and not losing the humor in the process.

There is an expression in Hollywood: Show me a comedy writer who went to the prom and I will show you a network executive. Being a successful writer was the first time I felt like I belonged. But even then I stayed a bit on the outside, as I was pretty sure that eventually they too would toss me out.

During the many years I was not able to own my unhappiness, my behavior was a big indicator. I have been a lifetime spiritual seeker, starting with an obsession with the comic strip "Peanuts" and the great life wisdom of Charlie Brown. In my teens I devoured everything from the self-help sections of newspapers to the writings of Hugh Prather, M. Scott Peck, and Alan Watts. (FYI, the last two have their own issues with alcohol.)

I've spent decades as a serial religion tester. Born a Jew and raised a Christian (a baptized Episcopalian), I have dabbled in everything from Hinduism and Buddhism to the First Church of Religious Science, in which I spent three years studying to be a practitioner. My home is littered with so many different deities, it looks like an eighth-grade theology class share-your-faith day.

I am one of those people who sees God in many things. I can sometimes feel the soul of my long-deceased grandfather in a bird. A full moon brings out a heartfelt prayer in me. And the more shallow side of my personality asks: How can there not be a God when you find jeans that fit you perfectly?

And that brings us to the subject of this book. I have always been a bit jealous of my friends in the program. I'm not in any way minimizing the suffering they had to go through to get there. I'm just jealous of the foundation that the principles of recovery gave them: The daily steps they had to live by are the most compelling and workable combination of belief, right action, self-awareness, and responsibility that I know of.

I have watched so many people I care about literally lift themselves from the proverbial gutter into a state of bliss and productivity. People who I thought were down for the count were suddenly at the peak of their game and living life in ways they never thought possible.

So I've spent some time over the years wondering: If it works so well for them, why can't it work for those of us who have problems—real problems—that just don't happen to be classified as addictions? Although I might argue that we are all addicts of some sort or another.

In an e-mail I wrote to Paul in 2002, I say, "I'm a huge believer in AA. I feel this would be a better country if AA or at least a program that dealt with the fundamental principles of it were mandatory for all people. Who can't benefit from being required to take control of their behavior and embrace some non-dogmatic, non-judgmental higher power?"

Twelve years later I feel even more strongly about that. I don't just want to be involved in the creation of this book and bringing these healing principles to a larger group of society. I want to *read* this book.

And I hope in its pages you can find some solace, some guidelines, and a way to get through your days and your crisis—be they self-generated or not of your asking—that gives you the same peace and comfort it has been giving those with addiction for over seventy-nine years.

Life is a blessing. As Paul has taught me to do, turn your compass from fear and loathing to gratitude and trust, and there is no limit to where it will take you.

—*Tracey Jackson*

1.

Shopping List of Bad Behavior

Somewhere in Here You
Will Recognize Someone
You Know: YOU

Yesterday I was clever

So I wanted to change the world.

Today I am wise

So I am changing myself.

—RUMI

Your Path

1. "I'VE GOT A PROBLEM."

Say it loud. Say it clearly. Close the door if you don't want anyone to hear you. Admitting you have a problem is the first stop on the high-functioning express: If you don't own it, you can't fix it. So before you do anything else, make this declaration, be it on paper, in front of the mirror, or as a mantra you repeat to yourself.

2. IDENTIFY YOUR PROBLEM.

Before you can begin to change your behavior, you must know what it is you're changing. We've isolated many common problems in this chapter; one or several may be yours.

3. HOW IS YOUR BEHAVIOR AFFECTING YOUR LIFE?

How do we know when our maladaptive behaviors have crossed the line? We often don't. And we usually have a well-worn list of excuses for how they haven't. We've included a questionnaire in this chapter that will tell you if your "issues" have grown to unacceptable proportions. If you're reading this, we're guessing they have.

4. ACCEPT THE FACT THAT THE TIME FOR CHANGE IS NOW.

The time has come to commit to a better way of living. "Soon" is not a time. "After Thanksgiving" is not a time. "After I've finished my exams" is not a time. Now is a time. Look at your watch. Write down what time it is. Write down the date. This is the moment your new life has begun.

W e are all human, thus we all make mistakes. Many of us make the same mistakes over and over and over again. In fact, we seldom make new ones because bad habits are just the repetition of mistakes, be they conscious or unconscious. Addiction enters our lives when we let the momentary pleasure or pain avoidance of those habits hijack our critical thinking and affect our behavior in ways that are either life threatening or life limiting. "Addiction," "bad habits," "poor life choices"—call them what you will: They all fall under the heading of "Lack of Impulse Control."

Do you talk about something you never get around to doing? Do you make grandiose, life-changing plans you never end up realizing? Do you find yourself saying, "This is my last [fill in the blank]": My last cheeseburger. My last affair with a married man. My last charge on my already overused credit cards. My last lie to Mom, Dad, myself. The last time I do not do what I promise myself I will. "Tomorrow I start over." "New leaf." "Never again." "One more time and that's it." Are you a member of the "I'll start tomorrow" club but tomorrow never comes? Are you easily derailed by the opinion of others? Does your own fear-based thinking hold you back? Does the idea of staying where you are, no matter how uncomfortable, make you feel safer than moving toward something that might actually make you happy? Are you ignoring any signs of danger ahead?

The advantage (if you can call it that) that addicts have is that they have their identifiable addictions. Whether you are an alcoholic, a drug addict, a compulsive gambler, or an uncontrollable overeater, you know what you are fighting. But if you are a woman who makes poor love choices, a serial philanderer, someone who sabotages friendships in the workplace by gossiping, someone whose go-to emotion is fear, or someone whose neediness drives people away, there is a good chance you have remained blissfully unaware of your addiction until significant damage has been done. The saddest wake-up call of all is the news that your actions have brought damaging turbulence into your daily life and more often than not the lives of others. Most likely, none of you are lacking for concerned friends or family members who are more than willing to act as human billboards reminding you of where you fall short. You screw up, the wife points out why, you turn to her with a look of intense gratitude and say, "Thank God you were there, Cindy. I never noticed. THAT won't happen again!" Meanwhile, back in real life, we know that seldom happens. More often than not, the repeated complaints of partners, lovers, and friends only drive us deeper into our cave of "Honor thy cravings; screw the rest of the world." Addiction is a powerful foe.

. . .

So it may be an unwelcome revelation, but awakening to the fact that the fly in the ointment is *you* is the beginning of change. The truth is at your door, and with it, the possibility of a new beginning.

PAUL

In the world of recovery, "First things first" has become something of a holy commandment. There's a reason such statements become bumper stickers. They're necessary elements to a proper beginning.

Addiction is in fact a primary disease, meaning it is not a symptom of another disorder. It must be dealt with before any of life's other challenges can be met. Whatever your personal disorder or dysfunction may be, if you are beginning your own path of recovery, the same sense of priorities will serve you best. Deal with your problem. There's no time like the present.

So what does it take to get us to walk away from stagnant, chronic, destructive behavior? A "Doesn't work now; never really did" pattern that has become a habit?

If you're not doing a single thing but reading this chapter, then you're already taking a positive step. That's because change begins with the will to change, and finding the will to change is a major triumph. Drug addicts become sick and tired of being sick and tired. Sometimes that's enough: the reality of change or die. For the non–life-threatening but life-limiting conditions, the stakes may be smaller but the rewards of change are large. Just the commitment to change, followed by those first attempts at a more constructive behavior, can be comforting. You'll be energized by the thought of a new and better life, one that is free of the daily "Oh, no! Not again!" moments after vowing to fix things "this time." So that said, let's get started.

TRACEY
....

In society, we are encouraged to hide our problems and cover up our shame. In the world of recovery, people are applauded for owning their failures.

Identify Your Problem

If one gathered together twenty-five random people and made them all stand up and talk about the problems in their lives, every one of them would have made a bad love choice, sabotaged an opportunity, hurt someone while defending their own position, or worried about not being able to control their weight, their temper, their lust for the girl or boy next door. We all have a laundry list of things we have done or continue to do that we are ashamed of and would like to change.

But before you can change anything, especially something that is most likely harbored in your subconscious, you have to be able to identify it. Let's start at the top:

The Seven Deadly Sins

Wrath, greed, sloth, pride, lust, envy, and gluttony may look like eternal damnation to a Catholic priest, but for some of us they're just a nice way to spend the weekend. I'll have lust and gluttony to start, with a side of greed!

While you may not feel your behavior can be described in such singularly biblical terms, chances are good that if you take some of your, shall we say, "issues" and break them down, most likely they will contain elements of this iconic group.

Let's start with **wrath**. Someone nabs your parking spot and the first thing out of your mouth is a remark about the other person's maternal parent, followed by a sexual slur? Road rage? Short-tempered with the kids? Boss always pissing you off? Actually, these days everything pisses you off. If that sounds about right, you might have anger issues. Sure, sometimes these feelings can be legitimate, but they still make you a card-carrying member of the Seven Deadly Sin Society. Is "I'll do it later" the first thing that comes out of your mouth when a task is presented to you? Is a job half done as acceptable to you as a job well done? Is your house a mess? Your checkbook unbalanced? Your résumé not up-to-date? Sounds like **sloth**. If for you there is any truth to the claim that the average male thinks about sex once a minute, **lust** is the runaway lead in your Issues to Be Dealt

With Department. Same goes for if you're a woman. Lust is one of society's biggest problems. From porn addiction to serial philandering to sexting—thanks to modern technology, what once might have been a weekly romp in the Motel 6 has taken on colossal daily devotion. But lust comes in many forms, especially when it comes to our stuff, like your neighbor's car or swimming pool. But we guess we'll be moving on to **envy** with that one, which is really just the marriage of lust and **greed**. Obsessing over your coworker's iPad mini? That's envy. Over your coworker's fiancé? Well, that's lust, envy, and greed all rolled up into one. Supersize me one more time—give me a G for **gluttony**!

You get the idea.

What Exactly *Is* Your Problem?

Don't even try and say you don't have one. We all do. You need to give your problem a label. We use labels for a reason: to let us know what's what. Without labels we would pour tomato soup on our cereal instead of milk, and pour Drano into the washing machine.

To help you find the right label, let's have a look at the granddaddy of shopping lists of bad behavior: "The Seven Deadly Sins."

How Is Your Problem Affecting Your Life?

Everyone feels these things from time to time. And they are by no means entirely bad or destructive. It's when they start to interfere with your life in a disruptive manner that they must be dealt with.

How do we know when our maladaptive behaviors have crossed the line from the occasional guest appearance to starring in and ruining the show?

For alcoholics and drug addicts there is a simple twelve-question test developed by Dr. Robert Siegler that is used to separate the social or problem drinker from the alcoholic. While some of the questions are directly related to alcohol abuse, there are several questions that might help you assess the extent of your own dysfunction.

1. Do you lose time from work due to your behavior?

2. Is your love life suffering due to your behavior?

3. Is your behavior making your home life unhappy?

4. Is your behavior affecting your reputation?

5. Have you gotten into financial difficulties as a result of your behavior?

6. Do you turn to disreputable companions and an inferior environment due to your behavior?

7. Does your behavior make you careless of your family's welfare?

8. Has your ambition decreased as a result of your behavior?

9. Does your behavior cause you to have difficulty sleeping?

10. Are you less efficient because of your behavior?

11. Is your behavior jeopardizing your job or business?

12. Do you use your behavior to escape from worries or troubles?

And we will take the liberty of adding one important question to the mix:

13. Is your behavior affecting your health in an adverse or dangerous way?

Now, if you are living with your madness at a manageable level and would like to keep rolling along in that fashion, you don't need to change a thing. But if you're fed up with your revolving-door anger at life's unfair turns, it's time to look down the barrel of your discontent, own your broken promises, give up your often tried but not so true excuses, and begin to change.

PAUL

One day in my thirteenth year my father missed a turn and drove into an empty cornfield. An angry farmer ran up to the car, looked in the backseat, and upon seeing two frightened children screamed, "What the hell is wrong with you? You're drunk! You're going to kill yourself and those kids someday!" He was absolutely right, and I suspect my father knew it. Four months later he was dead. He died alone when he drove that car directly into the abutment of a bridge.

Thirty-five years later I was doing the same thing: driving loaded with my two beautiful children in the backseat of my car. Why do bright, well-educated, and civilized men and women ignore such dark truths and continue on paths of self-destruction?

At this point you may be saying, "Hey, wait a minute, I'm not a drug addict. I keep my booze to a minimum. I would never drive drunk. I make everyone wear a seat belt. I pay the rent on time. Keep gas in the car. Walk through the mall looking and acting like everyone else. I'm a version of fine." Then one might ask why you picked up this book. Something must be gnawing on the wires of your psyche. Something must feel out of place in your world.

There is a lot of information in the promise of this book: *Recovery is not just for addicts.* You might not have a drug habit, but addiction comes in many forms. It's what takes your mind off of the real issues. It's what keeps you focused on something else instead of the underlying problems. The guy you are stuck on who never follows through—it's easy to get mad at him, be on and off with him, rage at him or cry over him. But if you look at your life, was there anyone else who behaved in the same way? Maybe Dad? Are you addicted to the patterns of push-me/pull-you? Is your understanding of interaction with the opposite sex all about confrontation and disappointment? Is the controlling dynamic of your relationships anger, rejection, and conflict? Do things not feel right unless they present wrong?

Addiction doesn't necessarily imply there are substances involved. Addiction to feelings is a powerful force. Addiction to feeling inadequate, addiction to feeling superior, addiction to feeling like you are always letting people down, addiction to feeling like you will never be the person you want to be, addiction to your excuses for why things don't work out. "If I lost twenty pounds, my life would be better. I would have a better job, a better love life, a better apartment. People might like me more." "So," one could ask, "if you really feel that way, what is keeping you from just cutting back on what you consume and getting out there and moving around? Or are you so addicted to the temporary comfort that food provides that it becomes more important than the guilt and remorse about overconsumption it leaves behind?"

Also, never underestimate the power of habit. Habits keep us tethered to something even if that something is not good for us—even if that something is in fact keeping us from what we really want. The reliability of a connection so powerful and long-standing somehow feels safe in a twisted way.

One of the big barriers to repairing our problems is that we are terrified of what our life will look and feel like without this "thing" we have become so used to. The thing can be booze, it can be heroin, it can be sugar and fried food, it can be constantly having something to complain about, it can be anything we glom on to that keeps our minds and feelings occupied and allows us to avoid our real problems.

Throughout this book, we will be dealing with many issues that come under the heading of problematic, consistent, and thus addictive behavior. They're the things that often keep us out of the very places we want to be in and from living the lives we want. They're things that are learned in childhood, tendencies that are born out of disappointment, or they are just plain maladaptive behavioral traits that for some reason we can't seem to shake.

Some examples of these are:

The Rageaholic

You stand at the doorway to disaster. Your hair-trigger temper has the potential to destroy your life and the lives of those closest to you. In truth, if you find yourself acting out physically, immediate one-on-one counseling is suggested.

The Workaholic

Your life is totally out of balance but your defense is a good one. You're a dedicated provider. "How the hell do you think the bills get paid around here? Somebody's gotta bring home the bacon!" is your loud response when anyone suggests you slow down. Losers here include the family that gets so little of you. What are you hiding from that turns your office into your primary residence?

Emotional Anorexia

Somewhere along the way you learned your feelings did not count. Or if they counted, they were way at the bottom of some list. Perhaps they were ignored altogether or ridiculed. There are endless reasons why we stuff our feelings where we don't have to deal with them: Sometimes they just plain scare us to death. Our feelings are the most honest part of our being; by denying or stuffing them down, we cut ourselves off from our real essence. Which in turn leads to any one of the outcomes we deal with.

Bette Meddler

Are you an expert at solving other people's problems while ignoring your own? Are you an authority on everything but you? Do you give out so many of your "two cents" that, if you added them all up, you might make the Forbes list?

Alpha Infant

You need constant reassuring. Constant approval. If anyone in the house gets more attention than you, it's suddenly a war zone. Nobody cares about your feelings. Nobody understands. A baby on the home field, out in the world the ego switch is often thrown and the Alpha Infant morphs into . . .

King Me

That's the I'm-not-much-but-I'm-all-I-think-about syndrome. Everything is a gigantic deal. Mr. Big Shot. Many times a playground bully all grown up. It's grandiosity writ large, but usually a cover-up for the most insecure. It is often labeled narcissism and is a host for an endless slew of unwanted internal houseguests who then strike up the band and present themselves to the world in an endless parade of poor behavior and rotten choices. If someone tries telling you anything you'll interrupt with a sermon on things you know nothing about.

The Hibernator

Today's environment has left fertile soil for the hibernator to grow in. Eighteen hours on computer games. Days locked in your room watching every season of *Curb Your Enthusiasm* certainly will keep your goals and dreams in lockdown.

The Victim

Born to lose and ready to tell anyone who'll listen. Put on this earth to watch the rest of us have fun, you sit in a corner with an expression borrowed from the tragedy mask and wonder why nobody asks you to dance. You won't ask for help because it's too much effort and nothing works anyway, so why bother.

Any Porn in a Storm

The person with the inability to relate to another human being on an appropriately intimate level resorts to objectification of the sex partner. The net has made instant gratification as easy as clicking on a link. This is a digital dilemma that's screwing with your life. No pun intended.

The Chicken Little Syndrome

You're still amazed the world didn't end on 12-12-2012. And maybe even a little disappointed. Even the Mayans have let you down. You broadcast disaster to anyone who'll listen. You always know where the nearest bomb shelter is and are convinced it's only a matter of time before you'll need it. Your fear-based thinking keeps you stuck in Disasterville and the mantra you live by is "What's the point? We're all doomed anyway."

My Phone Is My Life

Do you spend more time looking at your phone than you do at anyone or anything else? Does your heart stop when you think you've lost it? Do you say things like "This is my life" as you hold up your oh-so-smart smartphone? Do you find yourself escaping the real world by playing endless hours of Candy Crush? Angry Birds? Words With Friends? Is the cyber world a more enjoyable place for you to spend your time than the real one? Escaping real connection to ourselves and others through the world in our iPads, phones, and computers is a huge problem. After food it may be one of the biggest addictions we have today. If you answered yes to any of these questions, you most likely need to get a handle on how much time you spend in cyber space before it becomes your only place.

Charge It

Do you self-soothe with a trip to the mall? When you buy something, do you divide it up between four credit cards that are all a few purchases away from being maxed out? Do all the salespeople at your local Walmart know you by name? Is every expenditure your last? Spending, overspending, indulging our material cravings, keeping up with the Joneses, the Joneses' neighbors, and the Joneses' cousins has become our national pastime. One of the biggest ways we sabotage our own futures, our kids' futures, and often the moment is by overspending. It has become so easy. Some people wake up at four in the morning and head for the Jack Daniel's; others turn on their computers and take a cyber stroll through Target, Macy's, or any one of the millions of online shopping sites. Never before has feeding the beast of buying addiction been so easy.

This is just a sampling of what might be afflicting you. Perhaps none of these may apply to you, or you could be a minestrone made up of several. It's up to you to start identifying what the various ingredients are that make up your murky soup. No one can do it for you. Only you can take the actions needed to make the necessary changes. *The best time to start is now. Today. This minute.*

Accept the Fact That the Time for Change Is Now

You can't live in Tomorrowville. If you're always talking about what you are *going* to do, you are living in the future. If you are living in the future, you can't commit yourself to the present. To deal properly with your problems, you must be totally in the moment. Because that is where your issues live: here, now, in your house, in your car, in your office, in your bedroom, in your stomach, in your heart, with you. If you are not dealing with your issues in real time but down the road, some-

where in your future, you are avoiding reality. And chances are it will
remain on your to-do list.

TRACEY

*"Soon is not a time." This is a statement I end up uttering to
my children on a regular basis. Kids are great procrastinators.
If you have children or perhaps just carry on hcad-to-heads
with your inner child, you might identify with some of these
conversations.*

*"Have you done your homework?" "Soon." "Emptied the
trash yet?" "Soon." "Have you cleaned your room yet?" "Soon."
"Brushed your teeth?" "Soon."*

The adult version goes more like this:

*"I will get a colonoscopy . . . soon." "I will stop hoarding
and deal with the fact I can't find the garage door through all
the boxes . . . soon."*

*"I will lose the twenty-five pounds . . . soon." "I will file
last year's income tax return . . . soon." "I will start getting
my résumé in order and take that Excel class down at the
community college so I can maybe get the better job I really
want . . . soon."*

*"Soon," I will repeat, is not a time. Today, this minute,
at 3:47 p.m.—those are times. To really make a change, the
best time to start is with a real time, and that time is* now.

So I Have a Problem: Now What?

As time and failure teach us, a declaration that is not followed by carefully charted out, relentless action and daily vigilance seldom if ever works. There's a reason: Nature abhors a vacuum. It may be a cliché, but it's a great illustration of why so many people fall off diets, keep smoking after repeated tries to stop, and continue to engage in many forms of self-destructive behavior that haven't worked in the past and won't work now.

When an alcoholic quits drinking and commits to abstinence, there is suddenly a large, empty space—a void in his daily routine. The bottle, once his constant source of comfort and relief, has been removed. Unless this self-medicating ritual is replaced with something different, the old behavior will reappear.

You see the problem? You've got to replace the bad behavior with something else, something better. If not, you're headed for one more failed attempt at change. And there goes another chapter in the story of your life: "How I Almost Did It."

TRACEY

One of the things I have always envied about my friends in AA is the daily meetings they get to attend. I have been fortunate over my life to sit in on a few open meetings. Not only is the ritual something that ties them to their vows to amend their destructive habits, but the camaraderie, the instantaneous feeling of "While we may have never met before, I know you;

*you know me, and not only are we in this together, we are here
to help each other," allows them to feel connected to something
much larger than themselves or even their problems.*

PAUL

*All those embarking on new life patterns need support. The
problem is many people around you like you the old way. Your
spouse who could also stand to lose twenty-five pounds might
not be so willing to support your new healthful eating regime.
Not only does he not want to lose his Friday night lasagna and
evening visit to the ice cream parlor, but most maladaptive
behavior loves company in the same way misery does.*

*Everybody has a jealous friend, a bloated uncle, or a
miserable neighbor who will find something wrong with your
idea before you've hit the first exclamation point of enthusiasm.
And he will instantly turn your bowl of gusto into a colander.
So if you decide to embark on this life-changing journey, don't
talk about it with those who will not support you. In the same
way people in recovery gather together to nurture and reinforce
each other, find those who will support what you are doing and
respect the pledges you have made to be a healthier, happier
you. Keep your goals within a supportive circle as you move
toward rearranging the mismatched furniture of your life
experiences that led you to this cluttered, muddy moment in
your journey.*

2.

Six Affirmations of Personal Freedom

Your Map to a Better Life

This chapter is the heart and soul of the book; it is your road map. These six affirmations will be the tools that hopefully guide you to your higher self and tether you to your center.

Your Path

1. READ THE DIRECTIONS FIRST.

How many of us buy a new piece of machinery, toss the directions away, and then go "I don't know how to work it"? These six affirmations—like that espresso machine/pressure cooker/snow blower—are your tools for a better life. Your path to change. They each serve a different purpose and can be used both together and separately. You will use some more than others. You may not even use them all right now, but you will in time. And, like any new set of directions, you should read them all the way through before you do anything. That said, they cannot be assimilated in one sitting. Print them up, perhaps several copies. Maybe keep one with you at all times to refer to. Above all, never throw away these directions.

2. "SOMETHING NEEDS TO CHANGE, AND IT'S PROBABLY ME."

This will be the statement, the mantra, and the act of personal responsibility that you will return to again and again. It will be your first stop when the going gets rough. But, for now, it is where you start the changes you want to make in this moment. Say it. Mean it. Say it again.

3. GO AT YOUR OWN PACE.

Not all people are in the same place on their path; we are all at different stages of our development. You might know exactly what your problems are and can write them forwards, backwards, and in pig Latin. But for others it will take more time. Move at your own pace. Work through the steps at your own speed but skip none. You need to master each before you can move on to the next. You'll zoom through some like a NASCAR driver but plod through others like an elephant. The important thing is to keep on keeping on. This is a nonjudgmental, noncompetitive process: You make it what you want it and need it to be.

The definition of the word *habit*, according to Merriam-Webster, is "a usual way of behaving: something that a person does often in a regular and repeated way." In the *American Journal of Psychology* it is defined as "a more or less fixed way of thinking, willing, or feeling acquired through previous repetition of a mental experience. Habitual behavior often goes unnoticed in persons exhibiting it, because a person does not need to engage in self-analysis when undertaking routine tasks."

You see, that negative practice that you go back to again and again isn't merely a quirk, a tic, or an occasional blip on your emotional-psychological radar screen. In many cases it's as much a part of you by now as your hair color—although at least that's easy to change. Think of your negative behavior as a semipermanent tattoo, one that is stuck on your skin but not etched into your body. You can get rid of it, but it will take some work.

You've undoubtedly made attempts, but you're stuck. Maybe you've even written lists, set goals, made promises. But everything you've tried so far has most likely failed. It probably feels like you're always taking two steps forward and three steps back, the dance of a life off-kilter. Or perhaps you've had a brief period of improved behavior and then stumbled, staggered, slipped back, or relapsed to what was familiar. Call it what you will, you need help. You need a blueprint to show you how to change your mind-set, which in turn will change your actions. You need a new routine to replace the old one.

The people who seem to have it together usually have some set of rules, a code of behavior, guidelines, mantras, koans, prayers—something outside of themselves that allows their interior compass to return to the right direction time and time again. Some get it from organized religion, others from sports, books, or good parents who set them up to succeed. Some people just know what to do, although even they get off course from time to time.

TRACEY

One of the things I have always loved about the recovery movement is the guiding principles laid out in the Twelve Steps. I feel the same way about Buddhism. Look at monks. Have you ever seen a stressed-out, pill-popping monk? They live on next to nothing. They meditate for sometimes days on end. They have their teachings and their breath to return to. Nothing takes them off course.

Six Affirmations of Personal Freedom

The six affirmations we offer are useless if you don't employ them vigorously and often. At best, they'll become lovely little sayings worthy of a needlepoint pillow. To make them effective tools in reconstructing the way you live your life, you'll need to make them as much a part of your day as your toothbrush, razor, or morning run.

1. Something needs to change, and it's probably me.

2. I don't know how to do this but something inside me does.

3. I will learn from my mistakes and not defend them.

4. I will make right the wrongs I've done wherever possible.

5. I will continue to examine my behavior on a daily basis.

6. I will live my life in love and service, gratitude and trust.

The only way to break negative, worn-out, life-sucking patterns is to replace them with constructive, life-affirming new ones. You can't underestimate the power of positive rituals.

The only way to break bad habits is by using a set of tools that will show you how to recognize the behavior and then replace it with a new routine—a routine that, if followed with consistency, will become your new way of life. This guided transformation begins with the Six Affirmations of Personal Freedom.

PAUL

Some of you may retreat at the sight of the word affirmation, *disappointed and convinced such New Age frivolity isn't going to work for you. Before you walk away, I'd like to share some powerful words with you:*

"There is a principle which is a bar against all information, which is proof against all argument, and which cannot fail to keep a man in everlasting ignorance—that principle is contempt prior to examination."

Though attributed to Herbert Spencer, these may in fact be the thoughts of nineteenth-century theologian William Paley. But the sensibility of the quote remains no matter who said it. Approach this work with an open mind and reserve your judgment until you've experienced the results. Let the power of your intentions work for you. We've all heard the oft-quoted biblical proclamation "The truth will make you free." Not once did I consider it a defense against self-destructive behavior. But it is. I know that now. To speak the truth and to believe your words is a powerful step in taking control of your life.

1. Something Needs to Change, and It's Probably Me

It's a powerful moment when you say it and mean it. It's an awakening, an acceptance of a truth that until now you've kept locked away in favor of lies, excuses, and an endless blame game. You've turned away from defending your behavior to admitting your culpability. You've recognized your part in the problem and are prepared to change. You're acting like a grown-up instead of just acting out.

> "SOMETHING NEEDS TO CHANGE,
> AND IT'S PROBABLY ME."

What's going on? What is it that you've had such a hard time admitting is out of control?

While there is immense power in recognizing the need to change, it will produce better results if you act on information. This will require an adjustment in your behavior. So how does one begin?

Sit down, take out paper and a pen or a quill and some ink, a tablet, a computer, your phone, or a chalkboard—we don't care if it's a stick for scratching in the dirt (though that may be hard to revisit). The point is, you've got to start listing some serious shit.

What makes you unhappy? What is missing from your world? What did you set out to accomplish that you have abandoned along the way? Where is your life deficient? Your work? Your health? Your family? Or if no family yet, why not? Are you holding on to past anger and blowing up at people in the present? Do you immediately assume everyone will either let you down or abandon you before they've had a chance to prove otherwise? When things are going well, do you make a point of doing something that will screw it up? Do you start things and ditch them before they have a chance to take off (or not)? Are you afraid of success? Failure? Happiness? Risk? It's time to start connecting some dots.

Who are you not speaking to? Who are you not honest with? What are you not being honest about? What really hurts? List the things in your life you would like to change. Where are the places you might be out of control? Are your impulses controlling you or are you controlling your impulses? If it's the former, you've found a perfect place to start.

Now list these things in their order of importance. (For example, being disorganized is not as crucial as an inability to curb your spending.) Which ones do you feel are really interfering with your progress? Getting in your way the most often? Disturbing and disrupting your family and your work life? Keeping you from the life you desire to live?

The list may look overwhelming at first sight, but don't get discouraged. Remember that you did not create these problems in a day; you're certainly not going to fix them in one.

You may be saying, "I don't need to write this down. I can keep it all straight in my head." Maybe you can, but you can also manipulate the images and words in your head. There is something about seeing things in black-and-white—or burnt sienna and yellow if you are doing this with a crayon on construction paper—that makes it real and tangible. This list will become your blueprint to change. It will become the guide to your slipups and the road map to your dreams.

Look over the list. Read it. Reread it. Tweak it as new things come to the forefront of your consciousness. Once you start digging, it's amazing, the things you unearth.

Through the years, the "bad breaks" and runs of "tough luck" may indeed have had their headwaters in your actions or inactions. Look long and hard at the worst of the years and the amount of time and effort devoted to your habit. The more succinctly you can connect the two, the easier it is to commit to change.

Now write down examples of where things have started off right, then run amok. Is there a pattern?

What is the link between your behavior and the indiscretion? Do you see a pattern of self-sabotage? (More about that later.) Does fear trip you up and make you revert to unhealthy ingrained responses? Do you turn to food, the credit cards, or the iPhone for a digital detour in order to sidestep what you are really feeling? And in avoiding the pain, are you just creating more?

And the big megillah: How does your family—your parents and siblings—fit into this scenario? Are you re-creating the details of your past in your present because that is what you know and what feels comfortable?

It will take you time to put all the pieces together and begin to rearrange them in a way that resonates with you, but the sooner you start, the faster the process can begin.

Change requires the commitment to change and a blueprint for how to do it. Iron Man–like determination or world-class willpower have seldom been enough to rescue anyone from addiction of any kind.

Burn Your Maybes

Back in the seventies I was given the chance to star in my own television series. The title song I wrote for the show was called "Ya Gotta Believe." The show never sold, although the philosophy in the song still rings true to me:

Before you can commit to a life-changing discipline, you must believe it is something you need to do. To coast along thinking, *Maybe I'm not really that bad,* or *Maybe I can just sneak a little taste of whatever on the weekends,* isn't going to work. You've got to "burn your maybes." To do that, you'll need to prove to yourself that a change is required and the time has come to get it done. That commitment requires some intense self-examination.

For years, when working with newcomers, I've employed a little role-playing technique that may work for you.

Get out that list of mishaps, bad decisions, and pieces of your past that make you want to move to a new town so you never have to face the neighbors again. Now become an attorney working to convince the judge that the person who created this list would be insane to continue the behavior. Look at that list and plead the case until that sitting judge is convinced that the need for change is real and the time to change is now.

Of course the opinion that matters most is yours. You are your own judge in this little drama. The point of the exercise is simply to erase any doubt in your mind that something needs to change, and it's probably you.

—Paul

2. I Don't Know How to Do This but Something Inside Me Does

The second affirmation is a declaration of alliance. In a sense, it is a resignation too: the "lone wolf" label needs to be torn from your psychic jacket. This honest, positive declaration accomplishes two important goals: leaving behind grandiosity and arrogance as you affirm the presence of a collaborative spirit within; and creating a connection with a higher self that will, given the opportunity, make itself known in the days ahead. That inner voice will guide you out of the dark dilemma that has begun to compromise your moral standards, nibble away at your character, and negatively affect your relationships. Left unaddressed, it will eventually eat your lunch, your dinner, and perhaps the rent money. Decades of recovery have proven that this voice is readily available as soon as you are willing to recognize its presence. It is your inner ally—your "higher power."

> "I DON'T KNOW HOW TO DO THIS
> BUT SOMETHING INSIDE ME DOES."

Declaring the presence of an inner ally who will guide you toward a successful outcome will provide you with an arsenal of confidence and patience that you may have never known before. It is a simple yet not entirely easy step to take: having faith. Pure, unadulterated faith. But it's that wondrous leap of faith that accompanies all courageous acts.

For some of you this may not be easy. It's not hard to imagine a certain amount of grumbling and mumbling of "Bloody magical thinking isn't going to do me any good." We beg to differ. The physical changes in one's blood pressure alone are indicative of an immediate improved health factor in a positive mind-set. To repeatedly state that some inner presence is protecting you is to plant roots in your unconscious belief system.

3. I Will Learn from My Mistakes and Not Defend Them

We spend much of our lives running from our mistakes, hiding them, covering them up, lying about them, and often blaming them on others. How often do you hear "If my mother had loved me more . . ." "If my father hadn't drunk so much . . ." "If my uncle hadn't lost the family business . . ." "If my fiancé hadn't fallen in love with my sister . . ." "If my tenth grade teacher hadn't told me I didn't have a future in engineering . . ." "If my boss hadn't passed me over for his nephew . . ." on and on and on? For every mistake or unrealized dream, there are a million places to lay the blame and shame.

But this old liability can be viewed as an asset. The big blunders of the past may not be something you want to broadcast for the world to see, but privately a good look at the dismal details may provide valuable information about who you are, what you did, why you did it, and what it cost. And it may, in fact, prove to be an invaluable tool in learning how to avoid the same old pitfalls.

> "I WILL LEARN FROM MY MISTAKES
> AND NOT DEFEND THEM."

There is a treasure trove of information in the mistakes you've made. Unlocking it is a big step in building the new you. Pretending they never happened does not do anyone any good. And justifying bad behavior will get you nothing but a chance to "screw the pooch" one more time. So let's put on our serious glasses and look back on the bad old days:

What are you doing that is holding you back, embarrassing you, causing you to lie to yourself or others? Whatever the destructive behavior is in its current, out-of-control, bloated form, it probably began as a trusted friend that brought quick relief to the pains of the day.

Remember, there is no judgment here. We are on the road to fixing things, and you cannot fix anything by blaming, judging, or criticizing. That includes judging ourselves. If we do that at this point, we might as well shut the door and go back to our dysfunctional patterns before we even unearth them. While we need to be responsible, we don't need to kick ourselves. Chances are life has already done that for us.

PAUL

There's an old saying: "If you tell the truth, you don't have to have a good memory." It lives in your memory cells complete and authentic. Keeping my stories together as I juggled facts, timelines, and impossible scenarios was exhausting. I'm not sure why I ever believed I could pull it off. But when you're an alcoholic, it's part of the landscape: You learn to lie.

I spent years lying through my teeth in the interest of covering my ass. Nobody was immune to my self-serving insincerities, manipulations, or hypocrisy. Loved ones were the closest, so they suffered the worst of my behavior. My wife, children, business associates, and friends were all victims of my inappropriate and sometimes immoral conduct. I served one master above all others: my addiction.

I'd gone from the glare of the limelight and the work it brought me to hiding in my bedroom. Why? I wasn't Greta Garbo. I wasn't some romanticized hybrid hermit à la J. D. Salinger. I was a frightened drunk struggling to hang on to and hide the medications that my disease demanded. And in the fight to maintain the status quo, I'd done massive damage. It was time to stop the endless denial and justification. Telling the truth plucked me from the assembly line of rationalizing and defending my actions. I could examine the wreckage, the path that led to the misdeeds, and change direction once and for all.

The truth, when I was finally willing to tell it and live with its consequences, became a magnificent companion. Once we pull back the curtain of our deceit and dispense with the game playing we can discover the hard-earned lessons that lay hidden in the damage we've done.

TRACEY
....

There have been so many times in my life when I have been
afraid of what would happen if I told myself or someone else
the truth about a situation: I would actually have to face it
head-on. But as long as I dodged it, lied to myself about it, and
kept it under wraps, it might just crawl off and disappear.

But real problems tend not to do that. In fact they usually
do the reverse: The more you ignore them, the bigger they
become. The bigger they become, the more of your psychic and
emotional energy they tend to drain and the more damage they
inevitably do.

We know this is not easy. So start with only admitting your foibles
and screwups to yourself. We are not suggesting taking out a radio ad
and publicly declaring, "I verbally abused my wife when I really wanted
to yell at my dad." You don't need to sport a T-shirt announcing, "I don't
follow through because I am afraid of failure." At this stage, this is solely
a private matter. You're simply seeking the worn-out, negative behavioral
patterns you're ready to part with. It's time to discover and discard them.
The world of change, while private in the discovery process, will eventually widen to include the world around you. As you change your behavior, you will become aware of the opportunity—and responsibility—that
lies before you. There will come a time to look at the way your behavior
has adversely affected your family, your friends, your coworkers, and
your loved ones and heal those relationships. If you are honest in this
assessment, the next affirmation will feel like a natural progression.

4. I Will Make Right the Wrongs I've Done Wherever Possible

Hopefully you now understand the origin of the wrong turns, poor choices, and failed promises that have littered your past. But while knowledge is power, in this case knowledge without action is meaningless. This is the point where you have to make right the wrongs you've done. It's your mess, and while owning it is the crucial first step toward healing, cleaning it up is essential. It's how you file these things away in the "Bad Behavior" folder and no longer let them hover in your life or the lives of those you have affected. Be brave and know that the road ahead will offer an easier and more joyful ride once you settle those old scores in a generous and honest fashion. Be charitable and open whenever possible.

If in the past you have damaged, stolen from, broken, ignored, or cheated someone, denying them their rightful share in some success, value, money, credit, or ownership of property; if you have acted cruelly—consciously or unconsciously—toward others; if your selfishness and unkindness came from being under the influence of a substance or your own grandiosity, you need to apologize for and repair the damage that you inflicted.

"I'm sorry." Seven letters and an apostrophe. If it were a tweet, you would have 134 characters remaining. Yet those eight can make all the difference not only in your relationships with those around you but in your relationship with yourself.

Nothing weighs more than guilt. Rid yourself of that friendless burden and do not seek to justify your bad behavior or minimize your mistakes. Never ruin a good apology with an excuse.

PAUL

Have you ever stared at yourself in a fun-house mirror? You move a little one way or another and your image changes completely. Time passing has had the same effect on certain moments in my life. There were incidents in my drinking and using past that I examined in early sobriety and quickly decided that they passed muster. They required no apology.

One highly productive but tumultuous collaboration led to repeated episodes of questionable behavior on my part. Initially I felt blameless, but eventually I began to rethink the event and realized I was wrong. I'd been arrogant, flippant, and unkind. I was probably intimidated by the huge star I was working with and my ego responded with unkind jokes.

I began to see my own culpability in the tension that had been so well publicized in my relationship with Barbra Streisand. We'd worked together on "A Star Is Born" with very little time to accomplish a great deal . . .

An entire song score had to be written in seven weeks. Expectations and emotions were running high. On television I made light of the situation. When asked by Johnny Carson on The Tonight Show *what working with the legendary star was like, I joked, "It's like trying to have a picnic at the end of a*

runway!" It was funny, but it was also unfair. Looking back, I
saw that she'd bent over backwards to make me comfortable in
her home. She had demanded the best of everyone around her
and spent little time congratulating anyone for doing their job.
It's what we'd been paid to do. She was not a bad lady at all. It
was time to apologize.

So I did. I picked up the phone and she graciously took
the call, saying that she understood the process and appreciated
why I felt it was necessary. In truth, part of me was thinking,
But you're no walk in the park to work for. I didn't say it,
but I thought it that day twenty-some years ago. I don't
think it today, though. And I'm pleased that I didn't
dilute my apology with a feeble excuse to justify my
behavior.

"I am sorry" is much more than a quick Get Out of Jail Free card.
It is saying to those around you—from coworkers to acquaintances to
those you love—that they matter, that their feelings count.

However, the words on their own do little good if not followed by
right action. How many of us have been the recipients of what sounded
like sincere regret only to be met with the same offending behavior
again and again? Often people say "I'm sorry" as a knee-jerk reaction,
primarily to get them out of trouble. Kids are masterful at this. Many
addicts are stunted in childhood, so they still do it as adults. But words
without action are meaningless. "I'm sorry I got drunk and crashed the
car" means nothing if two nights later a similar scenario takes place.

But "I'm sorry I yelled and embarrassed you in public" is swell if
the behavior is modified in the future and it doesn't happen again. So

the words are a start. They are the jumping-off point, but we cannot re-iterate enough that they must be followed with new, improved behavior.

As anyone who suffers from destructive habits knows, the list of af-fronts ads up. So there are apologies of all sorts to be handed out. There is "I'm sorry for what I did last night and most nights for the last seven years." There is "I'm sorry for one big thing that hopefully will never happen again." And then there's digging up the people from the past who were hurt long ago. You might say it doesn't matter, but it does. People have long memories, especially when hurt or humiliation has been inflicted. And while the objective is to offer amends to the victims of your misadventures, the greatest benefit remains with you, the of-fender. You relieve yourself of an unaddressed source of guilt and regret. Only by making the amends will you find the true worth of that simple action.

No mistake goes too far, nor is it ever too soon, to amend it.

TRACEY

My best friend from childhood was ten years sober when he died suddenly of an aneurysm at the age of fifty-one. I can talk about him because he is no longer living.

He took his program very seriously and was very attached to the amends step. It started to feel like he was apologizing to everyone he ever met. I said, "You couldn't have offended or hurt this many people." He said, "Who knows what I did when I was drunk? I'm covering my bases." One day I asked him where he was going; he told me to a town a little ways away from LA, where we lived. He was taking someone to lunch. It was a girl we went to grammar school with and had not seen in thirty-five years. I said, "Why on earth are you taking her to lunch?" He said, "I shoved her on the playground in the third grade. I want to apologize." "Do you think she even remembers?" I asked. She was into her sixth decade at that point. "It doesn't matter. I hurt her feelings. I remember. I need to tell her I'm sorry." This story made a deep impression on me. It made me realize it was never too late to make right a wrong. He didn't want to carry the guilt and he wanted to do right by our former classmate. He wanted everyone's slate to be clean.

The Indians have a wonderful expression: *Namaste*. Much like *Om*, it has become a bit of a T-shirt and bumper sticker slogan. Though what it means is "The God in me acknowledges the God in you."

One "I am sorry" that comes from a place of undefended truth and is followed by a legitimate change in attitude and behavior is a similar gesture.

> "I WILL MAKE RIGHT THE WRONGS
> I'VE DONE WHEREVER POSSIBLE."

At times it's difficult to employ this positive concept. People who've suffered your wrongs may be gone or difficult to find. The challenge logistics create in living this proclamation may make complete success impossible. Don't be discouraged. There are other ways to succeed. As long as you make every attempt, even if it's stating your case to one of their friends or relatives, you have at least owned your misdeeds and taken action to correct them.

What happens when the apology is heartfelt, the behavior is modified, the proverbial ducks are in their newfangled right-action row but the recipient refuses to accept it? They are stuck in the past and can only speak the language of the old relationship. Or they feel the wrongs against them are such that they don't want any part of what you now have to offer. Perhaps they remain mistrustful or, as is often the case, they would rather be mad than happy. They prefer righteous indignation to a new start. Maybe they are more messed up than you are and you never noticed it. Whatever it may be, that is not your fault. We are not responsible for another's response. As long as we do the right thing—as long as "our side of the street is clean"—we cannot be concerned with another's reaction. We can be hurt, of course—we can be distressed or disappointed—but we must release any self-blame. Part of moving forward is releasing the past.

For now, enjoy the process. Look to the past with a sharp eye for harm you may have intentionally or unintentionally caused with your behavior. Look past the act and search for those who suffered from your actions. Offer them restitution when you can, and if you can't, turn to anonymous acts of kindness. While difficult at first, it's a glorious habit to create. You will find comfort in the practice. Within the act of giving you'll find the power of change tugging at your core.

5. I Will Continue to Examine My Behavior on a Daily Basis

Some of you might be thinking that this is starting to sound like a full-time job. *Make a list of all my faults. Own every mistake I've ever made. Track down my second-grade gym teacher and apologize for hanging her bra from the flagpole. And then start turning my mistakes into lessons. Now you want me to look at everything I do on a daily basis?* Let's just say it can't hurt. In fact, it's a great habit to get into.

Taking a proper appraisal of the good, the bad, the embarrassing, and the impressive on a daily basis is a great way to keep your goals on track. It's a reminder to do the right thing when you might have done the wrong and allows you the well-deserved pats on the back as you hit your goals and start becoming more of the person you want to be.

At the end of each day, look closely at your behavior. What didn't you do that you should have done? Put those things at the top of tomorrow's to-do list. What did you do that you shouldn't have done? Do your best to honestly undo it as soon as possible.

If we look at our lives like a business—things coming in, things going out—this is all merely keeping the books straight. A business cannot run properly without some well-documented information about how it's doing, and neither can we, especially when we are trying to make profound changes.

PAUL
....

There is an interesting moment between sleep and wakefulness where I sometimes remember startling bits of my past. In the quiet, undefended by ego or denial, I am snapped to attention by some gnarly little bit of personal history I conveniently forgot. Like a lost bill that's suddenly arrived, my first thought is always I need to settle this account.

The trail can be cold when trying to track down some former casualty of my caustic remarks or callous actions. And while always rewarding in theory, approaching someone I've slighted can sometimes be less than welcoming. I've had friends assure me that I'd done nothing that required an apology. I once offered a quick and far too casual "I'm sorry if I was difficult to work with" to an associate who had to endure me in my pre-sober days. He flipped the lock on his car door as I started to exit his vehicle and said, "If you want to talk about this, then let's talk." I hadn't given the ritual the proper respect it deserved. I was dashing off a quick note when a proper manuscript was in order.

Counting sheep is productive if you happen to be a shepherd. Tallying up your trip ups and triumphs at the end of each day, on the other hand, is a better way to spend those final moments before slumber—more so if your goal is to vigilantly catalog and amend your behavior.

Your daily appraisal is an effective tool to keep your life on track and to repair damages as quickly as possible. It becomes a marvelous habit—some immediate corrective surgery to smooth out the wrinkles in your conduct. A little nip and tuck to remove the negative residue of a busy life.

TRACEY

In "the Program" they call this a daily inventory. It's an interesting process that makes the moral to-do list a priority in the recovering life. Think of it as checking your compass orientation. These days we all have it a little easier, thanks to the invention of the Global Positioning System. The GPS offers exact information on where in the physical world you are. But the landscape of the psyche is a little more complicated. A few degrees off course left uncorrected for any length of time results in your reaching a far different destination than the one you planned. You let a little maladaptive behavior slip one day, get called on it the next, lie to cover the mistake, get caught in the lie, and are suddenly looking for a job.

The fact is, though, there's only so much one can do in a day, and with all the distractions of modern life it's almost impossible to stay focused and Gandhi-esque. Mere mortals tend to get emotional and reactive. Recognize the damage done, do your best to deal with it quickly, and embrace these life lessons. With practice, we slowly learn to sharpen our skills and master the art of restraint of pen and tongue.

> **"I WILL CONTINUE TO EXAMINE MY BEHAVIOR ON A DAILY BASIS."**

A quick review of the day actually takes very little time. Some find it easier to work through this process by compartmentalizing the areas of their lives where they may have a history of missteps. A relationship review begins with a life partner, children, and family members, followed by a glance into the workplace. A sexual review may be important if you've been prone to improper flirtations. Did you send a tad-too-friendly e-mail to the woman you met at the conference last week? If so, correct it the next day. Finances: Did you spend responsibly today or did you indulge yourself? If you indulged yourself, figure out a way to make up for it and climb back on the budget wagon. Did you drop the ball with your health regime? Did the cheeseburger win out over the gym? Whatever and wherever you are trying to improve, this is the time to take note if you are hitting your marks or falling short.

On the self-congratulatory side, this practice is a useful way to chart your progress. It's a way to mentally recognize and record the strides you have made and will hopefully continue to make. If you want to feel better about yourself, it's important to acknowledge the ways in which you are succeeding as opposed to diving under the covers, cloaking yourself in shame and regret. Daily notice of your evolution is a proven way to help keep you on the right path. Progress begets progress. When we feel good about ourselves, we begin getting used to the way good feels. That positive feeling replaces the negative ones, and pretty soon good feels better than any old impulse indulgence does.

Feeling good is the gateway to gratitude. The better we feel about ourselves, the more grateful we are. The more grateful we are, the better we feel about ourselves.

6. I Will Live My Life in Love and Service, Gratitude and Trust

Gratitude—Thankfulness, Appreciation, and Gratefulness. Trust—Faith, Belief, Hope, Conviction, and Confidence.

If we have done our work well and turned our lives around, if we are now on the right path, if we are through with lying, hiding, dismissing, dissembling, denying, regretting, and acting against our greater good, then these attitudes and ways of being will fold naturally into our consciousness.

Gratitude is one of those words that slips easily off the tongue, but is not always the first emotion we turn to. For some it comes naturally, like good manners and grace. For others it takes work—paying attention to the good and letting go of the bad. It's worth the effort. With gratitude as your guiding force, there is suddenly little room for jealousy, envy, sloth, or any of those other seven deadly sins. They do not walk hand in hand with gratitude.

Gratitude and trust stand on their own. They are the essence of the well-lived life. They are the re-creation of the charitable acts that give us our second chance. Or third. Or however many it takes for us to get to that sweet place of redemption where we know we've been given something magnificent and it's only ours if we remember to give it away.

Gratitude and trust are both the end result and the desired effect of giving your life to the process you have undertaken. The gift is in the knowing that your past has been your spiritual schoolroom with its triumphs, tragedies, and mistakes transformed into life lessons. Be grateful for them being the evolutionary key to who you are becoming. Be grateful for the perfect moment of awareness you're experiencing right now. You have arrived at a starting point in a new way of life. You are grateful.

The next step is decorating that powerful emotion with an equally potent action: You trust. The glory of your survival and growth through the obstacles of your personal history tells you that the best of what has been will be again. You have been given a new life and you now trust that as the future unfolds in unimagined ways, you will be cared for. You will have what you need to thrive. You are a miracle living in gratitude and trust.

And the best part is that you get to keep that miracle by giving it away. If we commit ourselves to an awareness of our fellow man's needs and address them in whatever ways we can, then we can, as the Native American offers, "walk in beauty." We can live a larger life of purpose.

If you've been relieved of the heartache of your habits and turned your life around, you have been given a rare gift. And with it comes a large reward you now have the chance to pass on to the person behind you. You can offer them your hand and guidance. You are living proof that there is hope for the hopeless, that the life-limiting habits that once bound you to pain have no hold on you today.

Pass it on. It's an expression with more uses than getting the gravy bowl around the dining room table on Thanksgiving. Pass it on. Giving is the permanent roommate of gratitude. Give back, in any way you can. This does not mean simply writing a check, although checks do need to be written by those who can. But it's the actual doing for others, generously extending your time and your energy that constitutes giving back. When you are in the ditches of darkness, doing for others is often the stepladder out. It never fails: The high that one gets from doing for others is so much greater than focusing on what we think we don't have. The adage "It's better to give than receive" holds real truth.

> "I WILL LIVE MY LIFE IN LOVE AND
> SERVICE, GRATITUDE AND TRUST."

There are many ways to give back. So many of our problems often live in the land of Me First. They also reside with the concept "Nothing is ever enough." That is where the gratitude comes in. In those moments when we start on the road of *Why isn't it this way or that?* Or *Poor me.* Or *This moment is so not what I want it to be.* How about taking that and putting the proverbial positive spin on it?

Sometimes just looking up and being grateful for the sun can nudge us right back into the moment of contentment. Sometimes it's just looking across the room and being grateful for our mate and allowing ourselves to forget that he might have loaded the dishwasher backwards and filled it with laundry soap instead of dishwashing liquid. How about a moment of just pure gratitude that he is there to screw up the dishes? Give him a hug. A hug is a powerful tool that not only connects us but also leads out of ourselves and into the place of the grateful.

Are you pissed off because your kid hasn't cleaned her room since her last birthday? Does it look like she's taking up a collection for the needy on her floor? How about not yelling, then maybe taking a few of those things and actually giving them to the needy? How about making her go with you? How about being grateful you have a child who is healthy and alive? How about making her grateful in the process? And how about replacing future moments of angst and anger with gratitude?

Are you on the verge of road rage because the traffic hasn't moved in twenty minutes? Take a deep breath. Turn up the music. You won't be there forever. Be grateful you have a car and a place you are late to get to. One can find the most amazing ways to take the moment and find something to be grateful for.

And in those most difficult times—the ones where it looks like any hope of anything to be grateful for has evaporated—that is when the trust comes in: Trust that your higher power has your back. Trust that while it feels like you are being tossed into an obstacle course of never-ending challenges, there is a power outside of you that will show you the way out. It may not be in your time frame of now. But if everything turned out the way we wanted, the second we wanted, we would never need to call on trust.

Through this journey, remember that you are being flanked by your greatest allies, gratitude and trust.

3.

The Carpet Is Dirty:
Is There Mud on
Your Boots? Or, Putting the
Affirmations to Work

You Got Yourself Here; Now Let's
Get You Turned Around

Your Path

1. MAKE LISTS: HAVE YOU BEEN NAUGHTY OR NICE?

As we talked about in the previous chapter, these lists are what are going to anchor you in this process. They'll help you understand the link between your less stellar moments and the maladaptive behavior that you're leaving behind. They'll also help you see the connection between the excuses you've been hiding behind and the potential you've been keeping yourself from.

2. "I SLEEP LATE ON SUNDAY."

Whatever your previous spiritual profile looks like, now is the time to make every attempt at finding some connection to something bigger than you are. You need to be able to hand your problems to someone, and your neighbor does not want them.

3. YOU'VE GOT TO HAVE FRIENDS.

While your neighbor may not want to take responsibility for fixing your problems, a good friend is essential as a sounding board and as a human compass to set you back on track when you wander off.

5. OWN YOUR STUFF.

That is what you are going to do, again and again. We've said it once and we'll say it again (and again): You are going to take full responsibility for all that is you—for all you have been and all you are going to be. You will say sorry to those you have hurt by making amends. A-mend. Break it down: You are mending that which you have broken, including yourself. You will take your goof ups and egregious errors and turn them into your beloved professors.

6. SAY THANK YOU.

You will learn to be grateful for the good and the bad. In that gratitude you will find trust and the knowledge that the future holds miracles that will reveal themselves to you.

This affirmation is a declaration of accountability. After an honest, detailed assessment of your life, you will finally be taking full responsibility for the conditions you have created. Here's how to get started:

1. Make a list of the things you've done in your life that you are proud of as well as the things that foster shame. Dig deep and unearth your carefully guarded secrets. Go back as far as your memory will take you. You are making a road map to when your unhealthy behavior patterns started. Be sure to include the good things you have done along with the bad. The *Yes* along with the *Yikes, not again!* **A history of misadventure is an asset to the courageous.**

When Addictions Are Fun

I am a bit of a spendaholic. It wasn't an accident I wrote the screenplay for the film *Confessions of a Shopaholic*. I would have to say that, more than fearful thinking, weaving catastrophic scenarios, and reaching for a bottle of disappointment, this would be my daily addiction.

If there is anything in life when you continually say to yourself, *This is the last time,* you know you are an addict. And certainly, when it comes to shopping, that would be me. I have never gotten to the point where I couldn't pay the rent or buy my kids food, and I have been lucky for much of my work life to make enough of a living to support my habit. But I have maxed out my cards. I have had to juggle payments. I have had to borrow from Visa to pay MasterCard. And I have sworn time and time again that this would be my last needless impulse purchase. And I have woken up with a financial hangover and defended my actions, only to do it again the next day.

I would like to say I only shop to self-soothe, as I do shop to self-soothe: I find a pair of shoes more comforting than an icy martini. I do. But, truth be told, I also like to shop. I like to shop the way many people like many of their addictions.

The sad truth about addictions is many things we are addicted to are fun.

Smoking cigarettes is damn fun. It is. Anyone who has smoked will tell you. It's not so fun now that smokers have been reduced to leper status. But when I smoked, I loved it. Now, of course, we know smoking causes a host of diseases and is one of the worst things you can do. That does not mean it's not fun. It means you have to curb the impulse. I'm sure gambling is fun. I have never found it to be so. For those who can take whatever they can afford to Vegas or wherever and play for a few nights, I'm sure it's a blast. It's recreation and entertainment. But then when you suddenly have the family house on the table, it loses the magic. When you find yourself at the racetrack instead of work, it's a problem. But the point is many bad habits start out as fun. One or two drinks for those without a problem are pleasant; five a day or five-decade benders destroy lives. Recreational things are by their nature enjoyable. Sex is probably considered most people's favorite activity. But nine hours of SwedishCookies.com a day could wreak havoc with your life and does.

I guess that was a long-winded way of my saying shopping is fun. Of course it's fun. It's America's pastime. Head to the mall. Four in the morning, can't sleep, go online, and try and find those boots you saw in *Glamour*. There is no end to it. And it takes place 24/7 all over the world. Open markets, souks, bazaars, bead trading. Again, it only becomes a problem when it impinges on your life.

—*Tracey*

2. Examine the pros and cons of your behavior. Where have the cons taken over and erased or derailed the pros? Can you connect the negatives with a specific element or activity in your life? Can you identify which of your problems are the results of the identified behavior? For example, has your sexual addiction caused your wife to leave because she found the evidence of your indiscretions on your smartphone and your boss just fired you for banging his new assistant during the firm retreat?

Is the bad behavior something you're willing to change?

If so, you're ready for the first affirmation: *Something needs to change, and it's probably me.*

> "I DON'T KNOW HOW TO DO THIS
> BUT SOMETHING INSIDE ME DOES."

3. Make another list, but this time ask yourself: *What are the excuses I've used repeatedly to defend my destructive behavior?* In order to cease using them, you must acknowledge what they are. It's not silly to write them down. You will return to this list when and if you find yourself falling back into the habit of using these threadbare justifications. This is vital, as you are owning that there is work to do. You may not always know what lies ahead, and likely in the past when you have felt lost or confused you relied on your old habits. None of us has all the answers. But in the quiet and stillness of our being, we can find strength. There are times when we must hand over the reins of power and just trust and know that we are not alone.

4. Look at your spiritual history. Are you religious? Are you an atheist or an agnostic? Are you willing to attempt a spiritual connection? For the believers in a higher power, this will be an easier task. If you are a skeptic, it's time to introduce a little flexibility into your thinking. Retire the hard-core

nonbeliever. You don't need to believe in "God." You simply must be willing. Willingness: It is the highest item on your list of immaterial needs at this moment. If you are willing to believe in the *possibility* of some unseen ally or invisible energy in the universe, it will help you in this undertaking. If you feel this possibility is impossible to embrace, at least try and open yourself up to the randomness in the unfolding events of your life. If you can attempt to see the light where you once saw only darkness, you might find yourself allowing these events to quietly convince you that there is something out there larger than your will.

5. The miracle hunt: List exceptional moments in your life, those events or occurrences that you might classify as gifts. Moments you could not have planned, incidents of unearned or unexpected grace. Perhaps the series of events that led to meeting your mate, lover, or best friend. The time you decided for no reason to take side streets to work, only to find out that you missed a ten-car pileup on the highway. You are creating a collection of positive or joyful incidents where you may find an unseen hand or power creating good.

This is exactly what you are seeking to recognize within yourself: an unseen source of energy that can lift you over the hurdles of habit and free you from the bondage of self-destruction and denial. We'll talk much more about this in Chapter Five.

TRACEY

What if you're a card-carrying atheist? In fact, oftentimes some of the biggest complaints one hears about AA is the religiosity of it all.

We are not asking you to believe in anything you don't want to. In fact, it is quite the opposite. We might suggest curbing your Chunky Monkey habit or Hothooters.com addiction, but we're not demanding you go to church as well. There are boundaries here. We will talk about this later in the chapter "God Is in the Details, or Wherever You Want Him to Be." But for the moment let's just say we want you to believe in something—anything—out there or just in your gut. Just a warm feeling in your solar plexus can be enough so you know you are not doing this alone. Something, somewhere, that will comfort you so you don't revert to the old dysfunctional ways. Something, somewhere, that will make the truth more bearable and allow you to take it out of hiding and deal with it on its terms.

PAUL

We don't know why it works. We don't know why the willingness to believe is almost as powerful as simply believing. It just works. So dare to declare. Speak to reach the peak! Know to make it go. Forgive the bumper sticker sayings, but the point is if you can affirm and reaffirm in simple fashion the belief that you are not alone, you may begin to feel an actual presence. And if you don't, keep believing. There's an old saying: "If you're

praying for enough faith, you've already got enough!" So feel
the Big Amigo beside you. Jump into that greeting card
mentality of "Only one set of footprints in the sand because you
were being carried by your Divine Cohort instead of walking
side by side." Corny? You can live on such corn.

6. While your higher power is important, before you go any
   further you need to find your confidant. It's Buddy time.
   Choose wisely. If you cannot find someone that you can
   trust, proceed alone and continue your search for the right
   ally. More on this in Chapter Six.

> "I WILL LEARN FROM MY MISTAKES
> AND NOT DEFEND THEM."

7. This is the time to really look long and hard at our inventory of missteps. If you have avoided making that list, now
   is the time to do it. Our first response to our mistakes is
   usually to somehow distance ourselves from them, especially those that are the result of poor behavior that has
   consistently tripped us up, destroyed our dreams, gotten us
   dirty looks, doors slammed in our faces, reprimands, fir-
   ings, and perhaps even run-ins with the law. We may not be
   good at following through on our commitment to change,
   but we have a black belt in "It's not my fault because . . ."

Defending bad behavior is like sentencing yourself to a hamster wheel of wasted energy: It offers no forward progress. The goal is to take responsibility for your conduct right away. Mistakes can be our best teachers. They may be strict, but if we look at them honestly and without any defenses to separate us from them, they will be our guides to our best selves.

It is important to remember we are not our errors, our blunders, or our misdeeds. That is historically part of the problem: If we identify ourselves as our foibles, it only causes us to feel more shame and embarrassment, which usually assures us we will continue to perpetuate whatever we are doing that we want and need to stop. You are not a fat pig because you ate two helpings of dessert. Ask yourself why you're doing it. Then remind yourself of your goal. You do not say, "I had to do it because my aunt made it for me and not eating it would hurt her feelings." Or: "I slept with my abusive ex-boyfriend because I was depressed and the guy I just met never texted me back." Now, these may be reasons, but reasons and excuses are different things. Excuses separate us from the behavior. They put in place some exterior factor over which we have no control that somehow is the reason we behave the way we do.

So, again, it cannot be said enough: Own the mistake. Learn from it. Ask why you did it, then examine the reason. If you need to check your lists, this is where they come in handy. What sent you to the massage parlor, gambling hall, fridge, department store? What are you running from, afraid of, trying to squelch? Why is the immediate pleasure more important to you than your long-term goals?

Look long and hard at the list of your negatives. Look for patterns. Addicts and alcoholics find valuable information in their "prelapses." What recurring events have contributed to your habitual bad behavior?

Careful review will empower you and prepare you to defend against similar scenarios in the days ahead.

Take that information and own it; it's yours. The only way you can file it away in the past tense is by embracing it. You won't move on in life until you take your mistakes by the hand, accept them as yours, take the lesson that they offer, then bid them farewell. It won't happen overnight, but learning to make a habit of saying "Hey, it's my fault. I'm sorry. I will work at learning from this so it does not happen again" is the quickest route to being the person you are destined to become.

Except and Accept

The road to unrealized dreams is paved with good exceptions. We are all guilty of taking this path at one time or another. All the things we want to do, set out to accomplish, mean to fix . . . except . . .

I really want to get out of this job and start that little catering business. I think it would do well. **Except** what if I'm making a mistake? **Except** I can't find the time to look for a space and set it all up, and I would have to dip into some of my savings. **Except,** while I'm not happy in this job, it does give me security, another twenty years and my pension kicks in. **Except. Except. Except.**

Accept the fact you only have one life to live, and if you don't take a stab at your dreams, you will always live in regret. **Accept** the fact you may have to juggle two jobs and some extra responsibility for a while but if the payoff is doing the work you love and being your own boss, it's a small price to pay. **Accept** the fact that your fear-based thinking has only held you back.

Many people end up spending their lives in the black hole of exeptions because it's often easier and less scary than actually accepting the situation for what it is. Accepting your role as the writer, director, and producer of the failed parts of your life story is a powerful path to real change.

Yes, there will be circumstances out of your control. Yes, sometimes the universe sends a season or two of tornadoes your way. But in the average life, we end up excepting far more than we end up accepting.

Once you accept things for what they are and really own them and take stock of how they are affecting your life and happiness, you have little choice but to change them and move forward.

1. Make a list of all your unrealized goals. How many are a direct result of your fear-based thinking? How many "excepts" do you use as an excuse for not following through and how is this impacting your life and the lives of those around you?

2. Accept the fact that you are responsible for the inaction that is a result of this.

3. Realistically assess your abilities. What are you actually capable of? A proper inventory of your talents will allow you to separate fact from fable. Do you have the ability to deliver the dream you seek?

You won't have all the answers at first. At some point you'll have to trust. And move forward. Sometimes just moving in any direction, even if it's not exactly where you want to go, will at least get you going. And you might just end up exactly where you are supposed to be.

Accept in the Other Direction

While we must accept our own realities and not live out the fictionalized version of our lives and personalities, we must also take accept and send it in the other direction: toward others.

How many people in your life, from parents, spouses, children, and friends, drive you either silently or loudly crazy?

How hard is it for you to accept everything from the personality quirks to the downright unacceptable behavior traits of others?

How often in the name of either peace or years of habit have you excepted and not accepted others?

What price have you paid for this?

Mom would be much nicer to me, except she had a tough childhood: Her mom was never there for her, and her dad was unable to express emotions. Her disregard for my feelings and oftentimes hurtful behavior can be attributed to this. But while you are ladling up the excepts, are you stuffing your own feelings and shoving your needs to the very bottom of your emotional drawer? And what is this action costing you? Are you resentful, full of rage and sadness that weaves its way into the other corners of your life?

We are all faced with people whose behavior we have no control over. If we let it, it can color our world dark and murky. It can ruin days, years, and lives if we let it. In these situations we have to move to the place of "accept." We have to drop the "except" and accept people for who they are, and that means who they aren't as well.

The "Everybody has a bad day" mantra can give you a moment or two to allow the "This relationship is OVER if you don't change" train of thought to roll by. Allow a little time for the dust to settle and then reassess the situation. If you decide to stay, the housecleaning may be extensive and may include a fair amount of your own debris. The "It's a wonder I'm not a sniper with you as my parents" thought needs to be replaced with the realization that we're all, for the most part, raised by amateurs. Forgive them and end the advertising campaign that requires you to share with everyone you know how screwed-up your childhood was. The time saved can be used constructively to make new friends to replace the old ones you bored to death with your endless complaints.

Often in accepting the imperfections of others we can forgive their emotional and behavioral failings at the same time. We can accept that there are people and things over which we have no control and then, if we desire, we can hand it over to our higher power.

Sometimes this is impossible. Some people are just too much to tolerate and fall into the "Life's Too Short" category. There are many who are not going to change unless they want to make that leap.

But even in the face of that, you change by dropping "except."

You change by adapting the position of "accept."

And in the accepting, you forgive, then decide if you are capable of carrying on a relationship with this person. Hauling around a sack of resentment does nothing but slow you down and bleed negativity into the vital organs of your life.

You can walk away. You can make that choice. But not before you accept.

And sometimes with the "accept" we suddenly find ourselves deep in the land of empathy for the other person.

We might not be able to take on their pain or excuse them for it, but we can become more understanding and sympathetic of their weaknesses. In the end, once we accept, we move forward from a position of strength and/or compassion.

—Tracey

"I WILL MAKE RIGHT THE WRONGS I'VE DONE WHEREVER POSSIBLE."

8. The only way to live honestly and guilt-free in the present is by cleaning up the problems you caused in the past. You cannot take full responsibility for your behavior without acknowledging that people, places, and things have been hurt, dinged, damaged, or possibly destroyed along the way. Now you must trundle forth to heal and repair wherever you can. Again, you will need to return to the lists you've created. Pay special attention to instances of destructive conduct. Collect the names of those people you've harmed and the details surrounding possible injuries inflicted.

An apology and an amend are not the same thing. Look at *amend*. *Mend* is the most prominent part of the word. Your job is to mend what you have broken. Be it a heart, a car, someone's sense of self, someone's property—wherever your blunders have left marks, you must now go in with a giant eraser and attempt to remove and restore as much as you can.

As we discussed in Chapter Two, an apology without action attached is a hollow effort. Look at your history: How many times have you said "I'm sorry" only to repeat the very thing you were sorry for, sometimes that very day?

Now that your behavior has changed and you know where your sinkholes are located, you will hopefully no longer slide into them. You can hopefully assure those you have wounded that the future will not be the same. But don't stop at the apology; let them know that you understand what it must have felt like being on the receiving end of your rant, depression, aggression, or transgression. You can explain the work you are doing if you so desire. If physical reparations to property destroyed or financial restitutions are needed, you must make every attempt in your power to fulfill those responsibilities. If you don't have the money at the moment, then try and work out a payment plan.

If amends are done properly, they can start with someone as important as a child you walked out on, abused, or ignored for your own selfish purposes and then go as far back as a third grade classmate you shoved on the playground. Start with the biggest, most immediate offense and then work your way backwards.

Do not be surprised if you are not met with open arms or a homecoming parade. Many hold grudges, and there are some people you might have pushed too far. And then there are those whose hearts and minds are not flexible enough to accept that people change. You are responsible for your actions, not their reactions. Once you have done your job, it's done. Have no expectations and keep resentment at bay; those are old feelings and places you no longer want to travel to. You can be disappointed but not angry. You did the damage and now you attempted to amend it. So hold on to your gratitude and trust, as you never know what the future holds. The person may just need some time to adjust and accept, and/or you may need to show them over time you are not the same person you once were. For the moment, feel good about the fact you cleaned up your side and let it go. There is great joy and relief in knowing you have done the right thing, especially if you have spent much of your life doing the wrong one.

> "I WILL EXAMINE MY BEHAVIOR
> ON A DAILY BASIS."

9. The only way you can keep tabs on your progress or slipups is by taking stock of your behavior each and every day. This is important, as you are not only acknowledging your possible backslides but you are also congratulating yourself on a day well lived. We all need positive feedback, and we should take it where we can get it. If you have met your own goals and expectations, then a nice pat on the back is encouraged.

End each day with a quick review of your activities. Have you met your goals? Did you listen well? Have you been considerate of those around you? Has your mood been volatile? Did you lose your temper? Did you control the impulse or did the impulse control you? Spiritual vigilance is key to maintaining a balanced life, because if you revert to old negative behavior, then immediate adjustment is required.

If you in fact slipped up and there are apologies to be made, then do it ASAP. You can wait until the next morning unless the person you offended or hurt happens to be lying next to you. That is what is so great about daily inventory: It's like cleaning your house every day, so nothing ever gets really out of order. We can do the damage control before the damage starts controlling us and those we care about.

You can write down your daily inventory if you want—smartphones make all of that so much easier—and then, if you are working with a buddy, you can forward your findings and discuss with them. Or bring them to your group next time you meet. By keeping track of these lists, they become an ongoing study. By referring back to them, you can chart your progress.

Here's an example: "When my boss flew off the handle at me for no reason, I simply smiled and said nothing. Normally, my own anger issue would have kicked in and a fight would likely have ensued. That's five days in a row that I have been able to control my impulse to get angry."

Or the flip side might be:

"I was an hour late today; I need to manage my time better. I yelled at the guy from Marketing when he took the parking place I wanted. It wasn't his fault. He was there first. I was mad at myself. I will e-mail him in the morning and apologize. Better yet, I will go to the fourteenth floor and apologize in person."

The good thing about the observation above is that it connects the behavior to a former irrational response. None of our actions are isolated: If things don't feel like they're going your way, it's easier to blame the guy in the parking lot for something that was not his fault than take responsibility for your poor time management. And maybe poor time management stems from lack of self-esteem, substance problems, laziness, fear of success, and so on. You can see how it's a case of "The hipbone's connected to the thighbone . . ."

The items on the list will vary according to the behavior being modified. Over time, the objective is for the good traits to become ha-bitual so less cleanup is required. Eventually your daily examination will involve more "did that well" than "need to work on." But no matter where we are in our personal journeys, taking daily stock of our actions is a great teaching tool.

> "I WILL LIVE MY LIFE IN LOVE AND SERVICE, GRATITUDE AND TRUST."

There is truth to the adage that nothing quite gets us out of our-selves like giving back. It is proven to lift depression. That's because depression is often a result of isolation. But, ironically, depressed people often keep to themselves. People suffering from shame or lack of self-esteem tend to hide out, numb themselves, and give in to other solitary or destructive impulses. But volunteering and getting out there and helping those in need keeps us in regular contact with others and helps to develop a support system. It also aids in making friends and allows us to come in contact with people we normally wouldn't. It helps us feel useful and needed. All of these things in turn protect us against stress and depression, especially when we're going through trying times.

And then, when you are feeling good about yourself, when you have hunkered down and built up your self-esteem by doing the right thing—when right thought has led you to right action and kept you from giving in to your worst impulses—there is nothing better to do with those gifts than spread them around.

Living your life in service does not mean to give up your day job and turn yourself into a full-time volunteer. There are jobs to be done and families to care for and lives to be lived, but there are endless ways to give back. Find the one that is right for you. If you have kicked substance abuse, you might want to help others going through that. If you have recently given up gambling, you might want to go visit the elderly in your neighborhood and maybe offer to drive them to the doctor or help mow their front lawns. Okay, those two, gambling and elder care, are not directly connected, but the elderly are some of the most overlooked people in our society, and many suffer from loneliness and isolation. As we have discussed, most people who are suffering or have suffered from some addiction have experienced acute isolation. So how about reaching out to those who are also isolated? The marginalized and needy in our society—the homeless, children who live in deprivation, and the elderly—suffer from great seclusion and stress. You will find great comfort and a sense of purpose in giving to them in whatever capacity you can.

Give back to animals, if that is your passion. We know of a couple in New Orleans who serve by volunteering at their local zoo. They say it gets them out of the house and helps them feel like they are giving back to the community. And one of them is in a wheelchair. So if he can do it, anyone can.

It doesn't have to be every day, and it doesn't have to cost money. It's a piece of your heart, a bit of your time. It's saying, "I live in this world and it's my job not only to take up space but also to help others."

It's also nice at the end of each day, when you are doing your inventory, to be able to point to one thing you did for someone else—something that was not required of you. Maybe it's simply carrying an elderly neighbor's groceries from her car. Maybe you leave a little extra in the tip cup at Starbucks. Perhaps you leave work a half hour early and volunteer to coach the neighborhood softball team.

There are a million ways to live in service. It's quite amazing how, once you make the pledge to do it, things will miraculously appear. When your heart and your eyes are open to see beyond yourself, it is astounding what you will find.

Then, of course, there is the essence of it all: gratitude and trust. The word *gratitude* gets tossed around quite a lot these days. Everyone is striving for it, and there is a reason. In our world of "more everything"—life on steroids—the simple act of gratitude seems to have gotten shoved aside.

We all want more: more money, a bigger house, fancier clothes, faster cars—all the stuff the people on TV have and tell us we need to be happy. We keep moving forward in search of something, but that something already lives inside of us. And that something is, simply, gratitude. It's stopping in the middle of the cacophony of more and saying, "What I have is enough; I am enough; I am grateful for all that is in this moment, all that is me: the chances I have been given, the things I have done, the good, the bad, and the embarrassing. I am grateful for them because they have brought me to this place. They have been my guides and my teachers. I am grateful to be in this moment because I know that this moment is all that I have."

Being grateful is not a Hallmark card sentiment. It's not an insincere "I'm grateful for the birds and the bees and the flowers and the trees" (although if it is heartfelt, you actually are). Gratitude is, in its purest sense, living in the moment. It is being attuned to all that is around you and being at peace with it. It's touching the unknown power inside of you and knowing you are not alone and that you are being guided to a better place each and every day. That is where the trust comes in. In gratitude we find trust; they walk hand in hand. They are the soul sisters of enlightenment, acceptance, and joy.

It is hard sometimes to find things to be grateful for in the face of tragedy, death, or the loss of money, home, or health. But it is in those times when we are put to the test that we must still believe. In those moments we must still, if not be grateful, then trust. Trust we are not alone. Trust we can do what we have to do even if we don't know how.

> "I DON'T KNOW HOW TO DO THIS BUT SOMETHING INSIDE ME DOES."

Trust in the silence. Trust in the unknown. Trust that little voice whispering in your ear.

That is true gratitude and real trust. It is very easy to tap these feelings when things are all going our way. It is a much tougher test of our faith if we can keep moving forward when we don't know what lies ahead, especially when things are at their bleakest. But all you have to do is reach out, and with one hand grab onto gratitude, with the other hold tight to trust, and you will suddenly feel that warm wash of peace and tranquillity that comes in the form of pure devotion.

Conceive—Achieve—Receive

CONCEIVE of the simple fact that trust is a powerful source of energy. If you can agree to "fake it till you make it," if you can act as *if* you were a believer, then you are contributing to your success more than you can imagine.

ACHIEVE an open mind. Look for examples of good fortune in your life and the lives of people around you. There are countless stories of miraculous events that become part of a family's history. Reflect on those incidents in your own life when an unexplained opportunity or good fortune appeared.

RECEIVE a sense of wonder at what lies ahead. You may begin to sense the possibility of success in unimagined ways. Do not leap ahead to outline your future but stay firmly in the present and feel the change.

4.

Why It Works

Millions of People Can't Be Wrong

Your Path

1. HONESTY.

Make honesty a constant companion as you go forward in this process. Without it, you have no foundation to build on. Examine your behavior, adjust accordingly, and repair damage done. None of this works without rigorous honesty in place at all times.

2. ONE DAY AT A TIME.

Anything taken one day at a time remains manageable, doable, and nonthreatening. If you attempt to tackle your entire future at once, you will be overwhelmed and defeated before you have begun. Right action becomes a choice—your choice, and not a mandate. If you slip up, tomorrow is another day and you can start all over again. We can all manage life and change in bite-size portions. When you start to feel frantic and anxious and like it's all spinning out of control, slow down and repeat to yourself: "One day at a time . . ."

3. YOU'RE NOT ALONE.

By invoking the aid of a higher power and admitting *you don't know how to do this but something inside you does*, you find strength and comfort. The future and its moments are not as scary. Your burden is lighter and your ability to see clearly is heightened.

4. EXCEPT AND ACCEPT.

By training ourselves to stop "excepting" and instead accept things for what they are, we find ourselves in a new territory—one where resentment has been left behind, where our relationships are not burdened by expectations. When our actions are our responsibility, we hold the power. We are no longer at the mercy of others.

Your journey begins with honesty. One of the hardest things in life is to take that long, hard look in the mirror and see ourselves for who we really are. What is even harder is to own our part in what might be the destruction, hurt, misdeeds, missteps, or white lies that somehow morphed into giant lies that rolled over every bit of truth that got in their way.

We lie to ourselves about who we are and thus we lie to those we love or could love.

The lie becomes the truth as we see it, because to actually see it for what it is would—and does—require an entire redo of so many past events.

Admitting we have been wrong to ourselves and others is one of the hardest things to do. It's much easier trundling on in the land of make-believe: Make believe I'm happy, make believe things are going to work out, make believe I don't have any of the issues that are bubbling under the surface and then explode in so many ways—most of them destructive and life limiting. Make believe I actually knew and know what I've been doing all these years. Admitting we might be wrong and have been covering it up is much more difficult. *Yes, I am having an affair with my assistant. Yes, I have been avoiding my anger at my father for leaving me and taking it out on innocent people in my life. Yes, my indolence and fear of success have caused me, midway through the race, to idle in the slow lane even though I started out with so many plans.* The list goes on and on.

Telling yourself and the world who you really are at any given moment is not easy, especially because we march through life hoping against hope that the world will see the image and not the flaws. But to be really loved and accepted ultimately means you love me for all of me and I you. Only then do we truly feel seen and thus connected to others. So taking that first step into the land of honesty is the most important step toward becoming healthy, and the one that if used daily will sustain us and allow us to grow.

The big question, of course, is: How do you get yourself to the place where rigorous honesty is the only solution? Sometimes our turning point disguises itself as hopelessness. Receive it gratefully and believe it is your new beginning.

This is one of the reasons it works. The light goes off; you stumble around in the darkness until eventually you begin to seek that switch that will return you to the light.

You start with jumping or sliding into the place where the only way to move forward is by being honest with yourself and others and picking up a big broom and sweeping out the dark corners of your life.

"Something impelled me to go to the bookcase and take down a volume containing the Twelve Steps that have given so many hopeless people victory over alcohol. I reread them, sensing the tremendous spiritual power that is packed into them, and I realized that for years I had been making a mistake that I'm sure is very common—the mistake of assuming that the steps are for alcoholics only. Now quite suddenly I saw that the power contained in them could be tapped by anyone wrestling with a power stronger than self."

—NORMAN VINCENT PEALE

"I've often wished there was a place for people to go that was like AA without them needing to be an alcoholic or be struggling with any other condition other than the condition of being alive. So many people would benefit from the wisdom, structure and compassion that is available in those rooms. I'm glad someone has put into a book what's been helping people for so many years."

—JOHN N., LICENSED CLINICAL SOCIAL WORKER

> "I WILL MAKE RIGHT THE WRONGS
> I'VE DONE WHEREVER POSSIBLE."

Amongst the wreckage of our past we find great relief in the occasional opportunity to correct a mistake, right a wrong, confess to a victim of our thoughtlessness, and seek a way to make restitution. It's in the repairing of others' lives that we can often mend our own.

This works because you've tackled a lifelong problem one day at a time—not an easy thing living in the nanosecond generation. It slows you down and loosens the noose you keep around your neck. "Okay, I did it today; tomorrow is another." Sure it has that Scarlett O'Hara ring to it, not to mention a tad of Hare Krishna. But the Scarlett-Hare combo can take you to a place where you can allow the process to take over as you put down the stopwatch and end the immediate-gratification narrative of "If it doesn't all work out by Thursday, screw it: I'm going back to the old way."

> "Beyond this obvious audience, I believe the greater population of Buddhists and other meditation practitioners can benefit from applying Twelve Step principles. As I've probed the Steps deeper and deeper, I've seen how they illuminate my meditation practice; they are not just tools for recovery, but an archetypal spiritual path in and of themselves."
>
> —KEVIN GRIFFIN, *ONE BREATH AT A TIME: BUDDHISM AND THE TWELVE STEPS*

One day at a time is really the secret to most successes. Being in the moment is the cornerstone of Buddhism, which does work. If you need proof, look at the Dalai Lama. Does he look like a stressed-out dude? And he lost his whole damn country. He lives in the moment. So just go slowly, get through one day, pat yourself on the back. You're in a better place today than you were yesterday (hopefully), and even if it's not where you want to end up, you're on the road and you're paying attention. A little progress is sometimes more than you think it is, and sometimes just doing nothing but sitting quietly and listening for your cue is the most active, positive move you can make. Yes, not moving is sometimes the best move and that is why it works.

TRACEY

I find sometimes that even one day at a time can be too much to ask. I tend to be a speed freak, and I don't mean I take the stuff or drive fast; I tend to do things very quickly. I am a multi-multitasker.

I do five things at once, often at sound barrier–breaking speed. I talk so quickly at times I need a translator. People are forever saying "Relax" or "Can you repeat that?"

Though I might be getting a lot done, I'm certainly not creating a calm environment for myself or those in my path.

I actually forget to take breaths. How can I be bothered with breathing when there are all these e-mails to sort through, clothes to wash, work to get done? I find my heart racing and my head spinning.

The good news is I have learned to catch myself.

I can do my tasks slowly and deliberately. "Moment by moment, hour by hour" is the way I am always reminding myself to live. It takes a lot of pressure off and allows me to savor moments and events. Even boring ones become more interesting and less arduous when I do them mindfully.

And in the world of making life changes, it is far less daunting if we attack it in shorter time capsules; for example, if we tell ourselves, "In this moment I am mindful, alert, and honest." Then we move up to hours and hunks of days and eventually whole days. It also means that when we slip up one moment, our new way of being isn't totally lost; it's just lost for that brief moment in time. In the next hour we will start again and eventually we are able to sustain that for longer and longer periods of time. That's when real change occurs.

The idea of a lifetime commitment to change is too massive to even consider. But turning to a series of dependable, easy affirmations as a regime offers a way to navigate a single day of temptation and makes a twenty-four-hour commitment reasonable, doable, and—when successful—something worth repeating again and again until a day of recovery has evolved into a life of freedom from undesirable behavior.

I t also works because you are not alone. The ability to trust in a higher power, a comforting guide through the troubled waters of early transformation, is essential. By relieving oneself of the need to control every part of your life and everyone else's, you'll begin to find a quieter and easier path.

If you do nothing but throw your worries into the sea or mentally attach them to a balloon and watch them fly away, you are on your way to finding a higher power. If you can simply visualize handing them over to your dead uncle Ralph who was always there for you and saying, "Uncle Ralph, would you just deal with this? I'm going to work on me and stop trying to control the entire world for a while," it takes a burden off your already overloaded shoulders. It allows the doors and windows of opportunities you never imagined to open and magical things to happen.

> "When we say spirituality, we're talking about connection. People who are addicted become disconnected. And spirituality, as it's emphasized in the program of the 12 steps, is profoundly reconnecting."
>
> —REVEREND JACK ABEL, DIRECTOR OF SPIRITUAL CARE,
> CARON TREATMENT CENTERS

It works because you drop the resentment. There is no question that resentment, backed by some good stories to justify it, is often more interesting to recount than just letting it go and not carrying around a UPS truck full of all the injustices you've had to endure. How do you defend why you are the way you are without those injustices? You learn to let go, and in learning to let go you learn to forgive others. And in forgiving others, you forgive yourself. And in forgiving yourself, you're suddenly not angry, anxious, waiting for someone to do something really crappy to you, because then, boy oh boy would you hand it to them.

Suddenly without all this bad energy swirling through your head and heart, you are lighter of step, kinder to those around you, and less burdened by negativity. You're actually a happier person with a whole new energy cloud coming your way. It's a lot more enjoyable than getting hung up on your sister making out with your boyfriend when you were at summer camp twenty years ago. Or your mother criticizing your haircut. Or the fact that you married a deadbeat. Many do. Let it go, if you can, and certainly let *him* go.

So it works because the way forward is unencumbered by the excess baggage of regret, guilt, and self-loathing. We no longer defend old behavior but replace it with right action. And by taking responsibility for the mistakes we make and correcting them wherever possible, we lighten our psychic load.

This works because the combinations of belief, honesty, right action, forgiveness, dropping the resentment, taking that daily score, and fixing your wrongs as soon as you identify them leads to one of life's greatest gifts: peace of mind. Keeping your side of the street clean means you no longer crawl into bed at night with a laundry list of mistakes you made that day. No registry of regret to keep you awake. Instead you can drift off as you silently list all the things you have to be grateful for.

It works because gratitude and trust take you to places that fear, regret, resentment, anger, and lying to yourself and others keep you locked out of. It works because knowing who you are and dealing with it head-on is a much healthier way to live your life than making excuses and pretending to be someone else.

It is our hope that with the knowledge obtained within these pages, the stigma of your disease or destructive behavior will be reduced and that the choice of continuing the journey to a healthy lifestyle will be an easier one to make.

Just try it. If your life isn't working out, it's pretty safe to say what you've been doing thus far isn't working. And if it hasn't been working, then chances are it's not about to start.

5.

God Is in the Details, or Wherever You Want Him to Be

He's Not Pointing a Finger,
He's Holding Your Hand . . . and
He's Not Necessarily a He

Your Path

1. FIND A HIGHER POWER.
Part of the process—natural and easy for some, a challenge for others—
is embracing the idea of a higher power.

2. MAKE IT YOUR OWN.
Everyone must find their own form of a higher power. For regular
churchgoers or those with a spiritual practice in place, this will be the
easiest affirmation to follow. But those who find it difficult to accept
organized religion or even the idea of something outside—or even
inside—of us that is bigger than we are must embrace what is in their
grasp. This will be different for everyone. For some it will be Jesus
Christ; for others it might be a song. But find something that takes the
onus off of you. Find a way (if you can) to hand over the power when
you need to. The comfort in repeating and believing the words "I don't
know how to do this but something inside me does" will allow you to
move through life with much less stress and fear. It is the heart of trust.

3. "I'M NOT A BELIEVER."
For some, making the jump into the deep end of the pool of faith will
be impossible. And there is no shame in that. It also does not mean the
affirmations are for naught or unworkable. For the nonbelievers, the
"something inside me" can refer to the collective unconscious or just
the warm feeling in your solar plexus when you know you are exactly
where you are supposed to be, doing exactly what you are supposed
to be doing.

The miracle of faith doesn't come to most of us as dramatically as it does in the movies. There aren't a lot of "burning bush" moments in most of our lives. The ability to rely on something unseen as a source of comfort and power comes slowly and almost unconsciously for most.

We've just thrown these Six Affirmations at you. Hopefully, they are roaming around in your brain. If we failed, you may be rummaging around in the freezer for that crusted-over Cherry Garcia. Maybe you're affirming the good feelings that come from your old habits. Or maybe, just maybe, you are walking around muttering, "Something needs to change, and it's probably me." Your significant other or boss said, "What did you say?" You whisper, "Something needs to change, and it's probably me." Or maybe the sound is echoing loudly in your brain. It's yelling, "Something needs to change, and it's probably me!"

There is a good chance that the declaration and the actual actions might have a lag time. Don't beat yourself up. Obviously, the sooner you move, the quicker change occurs. But better to plunge in whole-heartedly and with sincerity with an outcome of success than a half-assed attempt that will soon be abandoned.

> "SOMETHING NEEDS TO CHANGE,
> AND IT'S PROBABLY ME."

Perhaps you're really motoring and you've already made your list of issues and you're checking it twice. Either way, you have earned the right to congratulate yourself. Sit with the thought for a moment that this time you've actually begun in earnest. You've taken a long, hard look at the way you've been living, identified the problem areas of your life, and committed to the process.

You're no longer outsourcing your problems. You alone are responsible for the wreckage of your past and badly dented present. The missed opportunities, lost love, bent and broken dreams that got tossed into the garage and eventually carted off to that Goodwill dumping ground known as your unhappy past.

Let's take a moment here for a quick round of pass-the-buck. Everything that has happened to you in life is not always your handiwork. The company you gave twenty years to and were convinced would keep you on into retirement did downsize, they let you go despite the fact that you gave them your all, and your all was damned good. The economic slump was not your fault. Nor was the downturn in the housing markets. Ageism in the workplace is not a myth.

Your father's narcissism, the fact that your grandmother didn't love your mother so she was unable to love her kids, your sister's sociopathic behavior, your brother's crystal meth habit that took the college money for his rehab, your ADD, OCD, and maybe even bipolarism—these were not conditions you asked for. Cancer, heart attacks, and random disasters that strike when you least expect them and snatch the people we love, sometimes way too early—none of this is of our making. The list of life's unfair actions is endless. And yes, we can spend the rest of our lives nursing, medicating, and indulging our emotional and some-times physical injuries in a variety of ways. We can, and millions upon millions do.

But at a certain point we are accountable for our lives. We can honor what has come before—we can acknowledge where it has left its mark, identify how it appears in our present behavior—but at that point it's entirely up to us to fix it and take full responsibility for our actions.

> "SOMETHING NEEDS TO CHANGE,
> AND IT'S PROBABLY ME."

We are in the process of starting over here so the past is where it stays and the future is where we are headed. But for the moment we are in the present and you're committed to fixing it. You alone can do it.

But not really.

....

"I DON'T KNOW HOW TO DO THIS BUT
SOMETHING INSIDE ME DOES."

....

Part of any recovery or self-help process involves employing the services of an advocate *majeur*, hopefully one with superpowers—the basic principle being that, by recognizing a higher power, we relieve ourselves from the task of controlling our universe and everyone else's. We allow for something larger than ourselves to light the way as we step away from fear-based thinking.

Ask anyone who is religious, and they will tell you they seldom feel alone. They feel connected to their God or higher power whoever/ whatever it may be. It's why nuns and priests always have that peaceful look on their faces. They are not flipping out if they don't drive the latest car or aren't dating the guy or girl of their dreams. The big boss never lets them down. They have their perfect job. They are in harmony with the universe.

But for most people a life devoted to God is not a possibility. We don't care where you find your higher power. The sole purpose is to trust in *something* and *something other than yourself*, because let's face it, yourself has not been doing such a swift job of this solo.

It's all about the peace and strength you acquire from faith, not about the size, shape, or name of the power you turn to. No matter your personal religious beliefs, there's power in that ability to entrust some source with invisible babysitter-hood and to choose a church, temple, teepee, or mosque to fill up your faith tank. *Source* and *faith* are the operative words here.

It doesn't matter where you find faith, but you have to find it somewhere. And for each and every one of us, that will be in a different place. The whole idea is simply admitting that you don't always know what is best for you.

Belief in a higher power can be found in a variety of ways. Sudden turbulence in midflight or an earthquake in the middle of the night is often highly effective. A great start, but it doesn't always last. The thing about faith is it has to be ongoing. Your higher power is not a locksmith whom you only call on when you lock yourself out of the house and expect him to show up and make you a new set of keys.

> "I DON'T KNOW HOW TO DO THIS BUT
> SOMETHING INSIDE ME DOES."

If you're a dyed-in-the-wool "deathbed atheist" who takes pride in your commitment to nonbelief, we respect you. If when facing that final lights-out moment you have no intention of changing your dirge on the way to the land of the Big Sleep, that's your choice. The good news is that the second affirmation ("I don't know how to do this but something inside me does") can still work for you. It can work very well indeed with no bowing or supplication involved.

TRACEY
....

There is a misconception amongst certain people that one must turn into a Bible-toting, devout Christian fundamentalist or a weekly churchgoing member of society in order to follow the steps of recovery. Nothing could be further from the truth. There is, in a fact, a chapter in the basic text of AA, The Big Book of Alcoholics Anonymous, titled "We Agnostics." It addresses the concerns of those alcoholics who fear that their lack of faith in a god or an organized religion may prevent them from successfully utilizing the program.

AA is a nondenominational faith-based organization. You can find your God, your higher power, whatever you choose to call it, wherever you want to find it.

God. We can drop the word *God*. Once again, your higher power is whatever you want it to be. When addressing that most supreme being, we've been trained to use the most stilted, formal language loaded with *Thees* and *Thous* and major on-bended-knee supplication. The word *God* is a real turnoff for many people. Eternal damnation if you don't do it by his rules. That mean old guy in the sky who will strike you blind if you masturbate. Cheat on your spouse and you will come back as a goat. No. No. No. We are talking about the other guy, or girl, or sparrow, or—if you are Hindu—the holy elephant-headed Ganesh. Prayer and/or faith are easier habits to create if you're not forced to wander around in a forest of *wouldsts* and *Thys*.

PAUL

Gloria was a tough old bird—a heroin addict and a nonbeliever. She learned that faith was key to her recovery, but she didn't believe in any man's god. She did, however, love Neil Young. Gloria decided he would be as good a higher power as any. She grabbed a paper sack, wrote Neil Young's name on it, and set it on the kitchen counter. When she had a request or problem that needed solving, she would write it on a piece of paper and toss it in the sack. Hand it over to Neil.

For her it was enough. Her life got better. She became a certified drug and alcohol counselor and for decades to come she would save many lives. I worked alongside her briefly and watched the toughest holdouts give themselves to a new life under her loving care. Eventually she changed her higher power to the ocean. She would often stand at the shore and give thanks for the life she had been given. I'm one of many lives she made richer. Trudge in peace, Gloria.

Another option is that the "something inside me" can refer to the collective unconscious, the cellular history of all you've seen and done that is just past conscious memory. We've all experienced that strange phenomenon of trying to remember someone's name or the title of a film or book, a fact you've known for years but are suddenly completely unable to come up with. And then, moments later, while thinking of something else entirely, the name pops out of the murky depths of your mind. Somehow behind all the buzz and hum of your current conversation and thought, some mystical memory team was thumbing through scattered pieces of information until magically, with no conscious effort on your part, the information was there. If you can trust that inner process—if you can own it in an ego-free sense, see it as a gift of your molecular and electrical whizbang inner self—then you just might be able to trust that power and begin to use it.

Faith in an unseen portion of your own being: It's as real as the inner captain that breathes for you and keeps your heart beating. Something inside you that you don't control, can't find, don't understand, and yet must be there or you'd be . . . well, you know. Amen!

I don't know how to do this but something inside me does. Your power lives right there, nestled between your kidney and your spleen. We're not even sure those organs bump up against each other, but you get the point. It travels with you everywhere you go and you get to the place where you can't separate yourself from it any more than you can remove your liver with a butter knife.

We find answers in the stillness of listening for our inner voice as opposed to the confusion, anger, and resentment we generate from yelling our orders to the great waitress in the sky and being pissed off when she gets it wrong. Stillness, quiet, and prayer create faith. It's the belief that although it's not here now, it will appear. And one of the big lessons we learn is that it does not always appear in the form you want it to.

Something inside me knows the right door to open, the right road to take, the right city to move to. This guy may not present like my fantasy, but something else is whispering he is the one. Faith often requires that we take a chance. A leap of faith, if you will. The dictionary defines *leap* as "to move as if by jumping." Abruptly switch to something. Jump forcefully. Most people who are unhappy with their lives often complain of being stuck. They don't know which way to move. Leap with faith. Trust you will land on your feet exactly where you belong. It may not happen the first time. Or it may require baby leaps that add up to the big move.

The end result of all this work is a "spiritual awakening." And the ultimate gift is freedom. In the world of recovery, there's an amazing prayer that asks God to "relieve us from the bondage of self." There's so much information in that phrase. The "bondage of self" offers an honest look at what you've done to yourself as you embraced your addiction or bad habits in a stranglehold. You've denied yourself the chance to move forward and learn. Your method of self-medication has given you relief from the problem of the day rather than allowing you to step up to the plate and ask for help or "Good Orderly Direction" that would allow you to grow, which would allow you to learn.

There's magic in the phrase *I don't know what I'm doing and I need help.* Use it often. You can't save your ass and your face at the same time, so admit ignorance when you lack the knowledge you seek. *I don't know but I'm willing to learn* will become your personal open sesame: the foolproof key that can open the door to the cage you have locked yourself in.

In other words, it doesn't matter who stops the bus that is about to hit you or who throws you the lifeline when you're drowning. All you need to concern yourself with is the fact that you trust someone will be there at all times.

PAUL

In September of 1989 I went to Oklahoma City to perform.
I'd been drinking and using around the clock for several days and nights. The combination of sleep deprivation and

drug and alcohol toxicity led to a complete psychotic breakdown.

The promoter was horrified and the event postponed till the next day. I played the concert and apologized to the audience, telling them I'd had a reaction to my meds, then returned to the West Coast, where I continued to drink and use.

Two weeks later, in a blackout, I called a doctor and asked to be placed into rehab. That moment was the beginning of my sobriety. Twenty-four uninterrupted years of a drug- and alcohol-free life began on that day.

Ten years after that, in Nashville, Tennessee, I was to learn an important bit of personal history. After speaking to a group of alcoholics at the county jail, I returned to my hotel room full of self and an excess of pride. I was a river to my people. A unique combination of Jiminy Cricket and Gandhi—until my magnetic key failed to open my door. Irritated and suddenly far from serene, I returned to the crowded lobby. Waiting at the front desk, I felt a tap on my shoulder.

I was suddenly face-to-face with the promoter from Oklahoma who'd witnessed my Linda Blair Exorcist spinning-head meltdown. He just wanted to say hello. When I began to regale him with news of my transformation, he interrupted and said he'd heard that I was "clean."

A recovering alcoholic himself, he'd been sober seven years at the time of our first meeting. His immediate reaction to my episode was to phone several other alcoholics and form a prayer circle. A group of Oklahoma drunks I'd never met gathered to pray for my sobriety. Was it the power of their prayers that led me to seek help two weeks later? One never knows exactly. But

I would like to think so. For me it's the proof of faith. The
strength of handing it over. The Big Amigo riding in and saving
the day. The healing begun by one man's generous act of
kindness.

So belief and trust in something other than oneself is required, but
that something can be anything from the long-bearded, finger-pointing
guy from the Sistine Chapel, to a guru or your hot yoga teacher, to the
ocean, or to your long-dead Dalmatian.

TRACEY

Having been born a Jew and baptized an Episcopalian, quieted
my mind with Buddhism and been mesmerized into a trancelike
state by the cacophony of Indian gods, I must admit to being
somewhat of a spiritual Sybil.

I believe strongly, just not always in the same thing.

I never get on a plane without bringing along a tiny icon of
the Hindu god Ganesh. Making a quick stop in the church
next door to the radiologist before my mammogram. Lighting
incense and ringing the bells on my in-home altar to assure a
peaceful day, or at least one where I can rein myself in if I
suddenly spiral into the land of chaos.

In the end, one just has to believe in something outside of
oneself. The heavenward look and the whispered request or
"Thank you" qualify as faith.

The hardest thing for a self-admitted control freak is the
acknowledgment that something out there knows something I
don't and that I just have to let it go.

*But who is that person, thing, source of higher power? That
is the point. Many of us don't really know. We're relying on that
unknown known called faith. But everyone likes a name, a
handle. If this is going to be your special friend, it would be
nice to call it something. It makes it that much more real and
constant. Paul calls his higher power the Big Amigo. His big
friend, the one who never lets him down. I often refer to mine
as HP—higher power or Hewlett-Packard, the big printer in the
sky that sends me the printout for what I'm supposed to do and
when I'm supposed to do it. If I follow the directions printed out
for me, chances are I won't make as many mistakes and lose
my way.*

Faith is the entity we turn back to when don't know what to do,
faith that someone will help us over the rocks and to a quieter place.

Unhappiness and the repetition of those things that cause it are
often ignited by negative noise, chatter, the committee in your brain
that is either whispering or shrieking, depending on the day. "You're not
good enough the way you are. You won't get the job/the man. You don't
deserve it. It won't work out so you might as well not show up. Eat the
donut. Hell, eat the box. Spend the savings on a kayak even though you
live in Kansas. Or maybe just quit your job, despite the fact you don't
have another one. You deserve respect and you're clearly not going to
get it, so you might as well let them know no one pushes you around
like this. Don't study for your tests, prepare for the interview, clean your
house, your car, your life—it's all for naught."

The most proven way to turn off those negative thoughts and voices
is to replace them with faith: faith in yourself, faith in the process, faith
that even though today doesn't look like you wanted it to, there is some-

thing else better ahead. Faith, unwavering belief that even though you may not know how to move forward, something that is bigger than you does. Even though you may not understand what is happening it will be revealed. Faith in your breath, in the sun. Faith in whatever you personally latch your inner trust onto at that moment.

Love and hate cannot exist in the same thought. Nor can doubt and belief. So pick belief. Choose faith. Whatever else you have been using hasn't done the job, so why not hand it over to someone else? Take that leap with the faith that your higher power is holding your hand. And if you fall, that same higher power will help to pick you up and set you back on course.

6.

Hey, Buddy-Buddy

*The Power and Strength
of Community*

Your Path

1. BETTER NOT TO GO AT THIS ALONE.

One of the cornerstones of the recovery movement is community. You not only need an inner ally, you need an outer buddy to accompany you on this road. It's time to choose a coconspirator.

2. FIND THE RIGHT ONE.

Just because you are close to someone does not mean they are the right person to help you on your new path. Carefully select who you are going to reach out to. We'll tell you what to look for and how to go about connecting. Easy does it.

3. A COMMUNITY SHALL FORM.

Ideally, one friend leads to another and that one leads to another, and in a perfect world before too long you have a group of like-minded souls who meet from time to time, using the affirmations and sharing their progress, their challenges, their fears, and their goals. Suddenly you do not feel alone and you have also started sharing the gift that has been given to you.

> "We're all islands shouting lies to each other
> across seas of misunderstanding."
>
> —RUDYARD KIPLING

You can certainly add "and ourselves" to Kipling's quote. One of the hardest parts of owning our poor habits is opening up and admitting them to the world.

We hide things—from ourselves or others—because there is some feeling of shame attached. It's the drunk hiding his bottles, the junkie hiding his stash, the gambler lying about where the money went, the adulterer lying about where he/she was and who that text is really from. The spendaholic tends to hide her purchases, sometimes never even wearing them, and the overeater binges late at night when no one is watching. The angry person always has someone to blame. One of the biggest problems with this, outside of taking responsibility and amending our life-limiting patterns, is the fact that it makes us feel so alone.

But just as there is so much isolation in shame and subterfuge, there is such deep comfort in knowing you are not alone, that everyone out there has some shackle of shame they are longing to rid themselves of. How many times have you admitted something you might be hesitant about only to be greeted with "I thought I was the only one . . ."?

One of the reasons we actually continue in destructive ways is because we feel alone, and the immediate comfort of whatever our fix may be feels like an old friend who is always there to distract us. Bad habits are not old friends; they are bad friends. They are the bully down the street. Or the troubled "friend" who convinces you to do something you know is not in your best interest and makes you feel awful about yourself. You need to run as far away as possible from that group of friends. You need to replace those bad friends, those bad habits, with new, supportive ones. That means finding people who understand you. You need someone to talk to, someone you trust. There is no greater freedom than being accepted for who you really are.

TRACEY

Ask anyone in AA why it works and they will tell you "the rooms," or the meetings. They will admit that oftentimes the rooms were the first place they actually felt like they were home. In those rooms, one finds the most eclectic assortment of people. You will find CEOs hugging sanitation workers. You will find hookers arm in arm with the clergy. Black, white, rich, poor, educated, illiterate. They are joined by a common thread: their addiction and their single-minded desire to get and stay sober.

Those two things are more unifying than blood, social class, job, affiliation, or status.

The two components that are a major part of the success

of the Twelve-Step Program in its many incarnations are the
involvement of a sponsor to guide the newcomer through
the steps and the availability of regular meetings to attend.
The result of these is a sense of fellowship that is the polar
opposite of isolation, a common symptom of alcoholism and
addiction. The comfort and safety of sharing your truths, no
matter how unpleasant, with someone who understands and
perhaps has fought the same battles lessens and hopefully
eliminates the fear, sadness, and shame. It makes people feel
like they are part of a club, a group, a family; they are not some
crazy screwups destined to hide and run from the truth their
entire lives.

If you are committed to change this time and you want to use the Six Affirmations to do so, we recommend the inclusion of someone you can confide in: a real buddy.

Camaraderie, trust, and fellowship are the cornerstones of any strong social order, be it a business, family, community, or religion. We are meant to be with others. We are social creatures, and by *social* we do not mean "dancing till dawn" but that we live connected to other people who care about us and who we care about.

One of the biggest problems we have in modern society, though, is that people feel isolated. Gone for the most part are the solid neighborhoods, family units, and connected relationships we once had. The world can be very much every man for himself, especially these days. Technology has not helped. Look around a table at dinnertime: Everyone is in his or her own cyber universe. It is not only the birds who are angry. Anger often comes when we feel the most alone, the least seen and understood. Anger makes us reluctant to connect and is a mask for fear. In order to eliminate that anger and isolation, we need to connect to something or someone.

If you employ this program, the first connection you will make is the spiritual one.

> "I DON'T KNOW HOW TO DO THIS BUT SOMETHING INSIDE ME DOES."

But even with a higher power in place, it is no substitute for a flesh-and-blood buddy. Going it alone can be a bit like playing handball without a wall. You need a real person at the other end of the phone, text, driveway, or table. Someone to meet for a coffee when you need to talk, amend, repair, or just vent. You need someone who is there to remind you of your goals, your abilities and strengths, and to benevolently yet firmly point out your weaknesses. You need someone who loves you for all of you—the good, the bad, the ugly, the lost, the seeker, the finder, the loser. And hopefully you can eventually serve the same purpose for them. But we are jumping ahead here. First we need to figure out how to find that confessor, confidant, coconspirator.

It's probable that your personal dysfunction or bad habit isn't something you've intentionally shared or discussed with many people. Perhaps there was the occasional confrontation or accusation that left you shouting denials and outrage as you ran for your life. But running for your life can have the opposite effect when dealing with a major social, medical, or cultural misadventure. While it may not lead to death as substance abuse so often does, your isolation and sense of aloneness can hardly be an asset in building a better life. How many friendships have you severed because someone had the nerve to present you with the real version of yourself—the one you thought you were skillfully keeping under wraps?

PAUL

I'm not sure why most of my friends, family, and business associates chose to ignore my obvious addiction to cocaine and alcohol. It's been suggested that when the workhorse is pulling his own weight, you do not change his feed. And the substances I was abusing for many years had resulted in a schedule that I somehow managed to meet and the economic rewards were impressive. I actually experienced an early attempt at abstinence that was sabotaged by a manager bringing drugs into my home and using in front of me.

There was only one true friend who dared to approach me with his concern. Chris Caswell, who I call Kaz, has been my musical director, piano player, occasional cowriter, and friend for almost forty years. In the mid-eighties he dared to confront me. Caring too much to keep quiet, he told me how worried he'd been. "You're in way too deep with the drugs, Paulie. I'm afraid you're going to kill yourself. I couldn't stand by and not say something."

I fired him. On the spot. I met his kind gesture with an immediate dismissal. The last thing I wanted was to hear the truth he'd been brave enough to reflect back to me.

Prisoners of habit are usually incapable of hearing the truth until they own it themselves and are ready to take full responsibility. So well-meaning, concerned friends and coworkers are usually sent into exile or responded to with a list of their own faults. But you—ready to take the big step and commit yourself to change—need exactly that kind of brave, observant comrade at your side.

That said, while the song "Someone to Watch Over Me" may be a gorgeous piece of music, it's not the anthem we're suggesting. You don't need or want a babysitter. In a perfect world, it would be someone who is one part Louis Gossett Jr. in *An Officer and a Gentleman*—a tough gunnery sergeant who takes no crap, who expects more from you than you expect from yourself, who can be relentless and in-your-face when you need it, and supportive when you clear the hurdles—and one part Mary Poppins: someone who is loving, accepting, and all-knowing, connected but not enmeshed, maternal but not clingy, an unbiased thinker but willing to hear the other person's side. She would be there with a spoonful of sugar to help the medicine go down (unless, of course, your issue is sugar addiction, in which case she would be serving up broccoli). That perfect person would be there when you need him or her, but gone when you need to prove your independence.

Ideally, you would find someone who has walked a similar path to yours and come out the other side. Someone with their own issues, yet with enough of a handle on them to know what you are facing. Someone for whom honesty is the best policy.

The chances of you finding the perfect someone are slim, but you should be looking for some key personality traits. A person with the ability to be honest and direct without being judgmental is vital. It's much harder to lie to ourselves when we know that someone else is holding us to the truth. We can expect that only from someone who holds him- or herself to the same standards. Understanding and empathy are what you need, along with reliability. You do not need someone who is flighty or inconsistent. Narcissists need not apply.

Known gossips, the insecure, and prestige seekers should be avoided at all costs. The last thing you need is your innermost secrets that are hopefully on the verge of becoming an anecdotal part of your past being blasted all over town.

So move forward with caution, but move forward swiftly. Take an inventory of those closest to you. Who do you feel the most at ease with? Who has your best interests at heart? Whose life do you admire? Who has been through hell and come out of it intact? Who is struggling but open about their shortcomings? There are many ways to seek and find your buddy, though each is as individual and unique as each person and each situation.

It can be your spouse, lover, or best friend. But the fact that someone is your spouse, lover, or best friend does not mean they are automatically the best candidate for the job. You don't want your enabler or partner in crime to be the one, as they may not be ready to make the changes themselves and will possibly derail you. Or if conquering anger is your primary goal, you don't want your number-one sparring partner to be the one you look to for assistance.

Buddies of your own gender are usually the best way to go. The added confusion and anxiety caused by sexual tension and friction can only distract and undermine the work that needs to be done. Therefore, do not pick that cute guy in Accounting you've had your eye on to share the fact that you are ten thousand behind on your taxes and have a little issue with shoplifting that was under control until that mascara found its way into your purse at Walmart last week. This will only ensure that he never talks to you at Starbucks again, and you could lose your job along with any professional respect you have earned.

Do not pick your ex-girlfriend because you miss her or feel your lethargy and inability to self-start is all her fault for leaving you. This is not a way to get her back. In fact, she might have left you because of these qualities. So find yourself someone you have little emotional investment in or someone you are not projecting anything onto. Once you have your act together and have decided to clean up your past, then you can go to your ex-girlfriend and apologize for any hurt or anguish your behavior may have caused. This might not garner you an invitation back to her bed, but it may clean the slate and perhaps some new friendship can develop.

The point here being this: Do not use this person to get yourself anything or anywhere other than healthy and whole. This is why selecting someone of the same gender is the optimal choice. Rules may be reversed if you are gay.

While the person a shade removed is more often the conventional choice in a recovery process, a best friend can also be your buddy here. That is often the first place people like to go—a place where they feel safe. And frequently our friends do know what is really going on in our lives. They may not be talking to us about it or they may have piped up and were shot down. Just be careful they don't have an agenda. People we are close to are often invested and dependent on us with our dysfunctions intact. So we need to find someone who, while close and connected, can be objective and discreet.

. . .

The key word when approaching someone to help you on this journey is *cautiously*. To share the potentially shocking saga of your
misadventures in totality at first sitting would be ill advised. A toe in the
water, on the other hand, prevents a full-body burn. Go slowly. Offer a
little information about the transformation process you are embarking
upon and perhaps share that there are elements in your life that you've
decided to eliminate and rectify.

A relationship of deep trust does not happen overnight. Give yourself and your potential ally a chance to build a bridge of trust. *But how
do you even build this bridge?* you might be wondering. The first steps
are always the hardest. Once you have identified your suspects, choose
several in the event they either do not want to be a part of your process
or they bail on you. There is also the possibility they could turn out to
be more screwed-up than you thought.

But even the damaged can be insightful and trustworthy, so if you
do find someone who fits that bill and your proposition awakens something in them, there can be a quid pro quo relationship where you wind
up supporting each other. This is often an ideal situation, as both people feel empowered and both feel needed. But there are many ways to
approach it, and ideally you will find the one that is right for you.

So now you have identified your first choice. For our purposes
we will call her Laurie. You have known Laurie for several years. She
is open and honest and a no-bullshit character. She remains centered
despite having to deal with ongoing difficult family problems and has
survived a sticky divorce. She does not blame others for her problems.
She is not your best friend; your lives do not intersect in many places.

You met her when you briefly went to the gym, before you gave it up. You had coffee with her several times and she encouraged you to keep coming to work out. You ignored several e-mails from her asking you to meet up after your next trip to the gym. But you were embarrassed when you let your membership go. Well, you are redoing your life here, aren't you?

The first step is to call or e-mail Laurie and apologize for not having responded to her invitations. It is never too soon to own your poor behavior and make right your wrongs. Without giving away your entire story, tell her you have been going through some life-changing events. You would love to take her to coffee and play catch-up. Keep it brief at this point; the way she responds will be an indicator if this is the right person to align yourself with. If she doesn't get back to you within a few days, move on. You need someone who returns e-mails and calls. Reliability is key here. In a perfect world, Laurie gets back to you the next day or two and you make a date for coffee.

When the day comes, show up on time. Do not make her wait. If being late is one of your issues, this is a place to start being on time. You treat—unless Laurie is an heiress and you are down to your last rent check. If that is the case, invite her to your place or meet her in the park with a thermos and suggest a walk. You are about to ask for a huge favor; you need to pick up the tab. If being a mooch is one of your problems, this is a place to develop new habits. The way we interact with our ally in this is the way we hope to begin interacting with the world. Show up. Be responsible. Own your stuff. Take control. Honesty rules. This is possibly the first time these concepts will become action.

After a little small talk you can see if Laurie is, in fact, your girl. At which point you jump in, albeit slowly.

"Laurie, as you probably noticed by my not returning to the gym, I have some issues with follow-through. You must have figured that out when I never got back to you. I want you to know I enjoyed the time we spent together; I didn't get back to you because I was embarrassed about not making good on my commitment. I'm actually embarrassed by a number of things. You might have noticed that I can present as a bit of a mess. [You don't have to say this, but can if you want to add a bit of levity.] And I'm committed to changing once and for all, which is one of the reasons I wanted to talk to you today."

Obviously you need to leave some space for her to reply. But for the moment, what you say is the controlling dynamic. Let her chime in. If she is scolding, dogmatic, or unsympathetic, you should switch the talk to something neutral quickly, and when the lattes are done, thank her and head for the nearest exit.

But if she responds with empathy and interest in what you have to say, you should keep going. You may have found your buddy.

Now talk about the path you wish to take.

"I have come to the place, Laurie, where I realize something needs to change, and it's probably me." Explain that you are preparing to make important adjustments in the way you live your life and that you're looking for someone to help monitor your progress and observe the change.

At this stage it's really important that you don't scare people away. You are not looking for a free shrink or a constant companion. You are looking for a buddy. Someone you can call when you need a boost. Someone who can hold you to the standards you are trying to hold yourself to. Someone you can turn to when you feel yourself sliding backwards and who will firmly but gently nudge you back onto your path.

The relationship between you and your guide is a hybrid built on mutual respect. It's one that will require a degree of discipline that goes beyond the normal "me and my homies" friendship. Choosing some-one is something of an endowment. You are elevating their position in your world, and as you open your intimate history to them, be prepared to receive their honest reactions. You may not like what you hear. Do not overreact.

Remember that the tempo of the conversation and the amount of detail you share will depend on the response of your candidate. If the person is willing to help you out, the two of you can chart out a game plan together. Or you can show him or her the affirmations and share how you wish to employ them.

Be open to suggestions from your buddy. If he or she is willing to be a part of your program, that person needs to feel like a participant, unless he or she wants a more backseat role. Again, this is all dependent on the individuals involved and the level of dysfunction that is being corrected. If you are merely losing ten pounds or trying to stop gos-siping, it is a very different scenario than someone with deeply self-sabotaging habits. The person with a long history of broken dreams and shattered life experiences is going to require some real monitoring. The serial adulterer or sex addict who is destroying relationships or other people with the speed of the Terminator will not shake their lack of impulse control without vigilance and diligence each step of the way.

Sharing the very deep part of ourselves that has been hidden and cloaked in shame with someone else is deeply personal; there is no one-size-fits-all solution. So while this may not sound as helpful as one would like, you have to make these decisions for yourself. Part of the process you are going through is taking control of your own life and changing the way you think, respond, and behave. A large part of that is learning to make healthy choices, be they about the people you decide to love, the work you decide to do, or the foods you choose to eat. This is about being in control and not letting negative impulses and outside influences rule your world. So one of the first big steps is the quality and character of whom you pick to help you out.

Once you open up and share your problems and the desire to alter them, chances are your buddy will have some personal cleanup work to do too. Who among us does not? In a perfect scenario you will in time become a support for each other. And then, as you feel confident and secure, you might choose to invite others into your circle. You don't want to do this too quickly. First you will want to achieve some success and confidence in your own transformation. But eventually, how nice would it be to configure a group of people who meet up for coffee, hikes, or potluck suppers where everyone shares their desires for change, their foibles, their fears, and works on their goals and affirmations together!

Over time, a tight community can form. It can be a safe haven where you can openly discuss your evolution from who you've been to who you are becoming—where you can learn from others on a similar path and share the truths you've uncovered along the way about yourself and the changing world you are learning to be a part of. You all have the freedom to own not being perfect, to slipping up, to making mistakes. Your stumbles will be met with good advice given without judgment, a hug when needed, or an "Oh, boy, do I know that one. I did the same thing last week." You can also share your triumphs, your fears, your dreams, and sometimes the disasters all of us face that are not of our own making. You can be part of a club where the only requirement for membership is a desire to change and to be purely human, without all the walls and defenses. The goal is to live and connect, minus the smoke and the mirrors and the projection of a perfect self that does not exist for anyone anywhere.

We all spend so much of our lives leaning over the fence, convinced the person on the other side has it so much more together. They have a better relationship with their spouse, mother, son, boss. They have a better job and more confidence; they don't suffer from addictive traits, late-night demons, fears that ride shotgun next to them, or destructive impulses that control them. They have better sex, smaller thighs, more love, fewer needs, fears, and bruises. They are some idealized, projected character that only serves to make us feel more embarrassed and unhappy with who we are. And this, more often than not, only perpetuates the shame and isolation that keeps us locked into the very corner we do not want to be in. The first step in breaking down that fence is trusting that you may not know how to do this but something inside you does. Owning that you are human and want and need change is an initial act of trust. Before long, one buddy will lead to another and another and another. Soon you will not feel alone, isolated, and misunderstood. You will form a base camp that will attract others and the fences will all come down. Be grateful.

7.

Weighty Issues

Even If Food Isn't Your Issue,

It Often Is

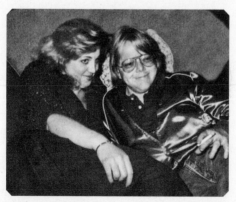

*Tracey and Paul thirty-five years ago. No, we were
not dating. We were on Robert Mitchum's bed.
Paul was drunk. Tracey was starstruck. We would
both get over these conditions.*

Your Path

1. GET HEALTHY.

Diets don't work; changing your lifestyle permanently does. If you want to be truly healthy, it's a lifetime commitment that starts now.

2. UNDERSTAND HOW YOU USE FOOD.

Do you use it to fill a void? Do you get the most comfort from comfort foods? Do you stuff your feelings by stuffing yourself?

3. IT'S NOT *WHAT* YOU EAT, IT'S *WHY* YOU EAT.

Create a Mood-to-Food Journal (which we'll talk more about in this chapter). Examine the emotional landscape before you eat. Note *why* you eat and *when* you eat. Your objective is to begin to see the connection between a negative experience and the use of food as a Band-Aid.

4. WORK OUT.

Just do it. Whatever you can, whenever you can. Join a group. Jog on your own. Find something you like and make it a nonnegotiable part of your days.

5. MAKE IT ENJOYABLE.

Make healthy habits fun. People cringe at the thought of eating right and exercising. Healthy habits are often considered punitive. Change that. Take your family and friends on the journey with you. Good health loves company!

Without question, one of the biggest health problems in America today is being overweight and obesity. To put it in perspective, 15 percent of the adult population are considered "problem" drinkers, while a whopping 68 percent are overweight and 35 percent are classified as obese. According to a Stanford Hospital & Clinics study, each year obesity-related conditions cost over $150 billion and cause an estimated 300,000 premature deaths in the U.S. It's a staggering sum. Alcohol-related deaths come in at 75,000, a figure that deserves attention—serious attention—but it's nowhere near the amount caused by the overconsumption of food. And the projected stats are even more alarming: A CDC report projects that by the year 2030, 42 *percent* of Americans will be obese. Add in the 68 percent who are already overweight and you have a number that basically includes the entire country!

While neither one of us would have been considered obese when you look at our photo, we both fell into the overweight camp. Between us, we have gained and lost at least three John Goodmans in our lifetime.

PAUL
....

I've struggled with excess weight for most of my life. I'm one of the few who got fat while doing vast quantities of cocaine. I'd drink and do blow all day and then, when the last of the drugs were gone, I'd empty the contents of the refrigerator into a saucepan, stir until disgusting, and then devour. Rising midafternoon, I'd wander into the kitchen and be amazed at the debris. At my peak I weighed 187. I remind you that I'm five-two.

There were intervals of discipline where I'd drop a few pounds, but somehow they always returned. I'd bounce around onstage, feeling all that love from an audience, and then return to an empty hotel room. Suddenly alone, I'd be in trouble, looking for something to fix that feeling of abandonment. I'd take one look at that empty bed and abandon any plans to eat sensibly. I have abandonment issues in more ways than one. A full fridge was often the answer.

Like the cigarette that followed
The ringing of the phone
I get hungry when I realize
I'm going to bed alone.

Making the connection between the emotion and the need has been key to my weight loss. Recognizing when and why I

ate has offered real insight to issues beyond just diet. The
"connections" are equal signs that I've used to turn my
relationship with food into a healthy partnership.

TRACEY

While I didn't drink or do drugs, I had a giant vat of loneliness
that I constantly tried to stuff with food, clothes, boys, and
more food, which meant bigger clothes and bigger boys. It
wasn't until I looked long and hard at who I was that I found
the source of my endless craving for food. It was a feeling of lack
in other areas of my life. Once I was able to get a handle on
what I was doing and why, I was on my way to getting it under
control.

I suffered from a lack of self-esteem that went back to my
childhood. My dad left when I was young and his new family
came first. From this and other things I was left with a feeling
that I didn't belong. Like so many of us, I self-soothed with
food. When I was fat, I would eat at the end of the day when
I came home to an empty apartment and knew I faced another
evening alone without anyone to spend time with. Would this
be the way the rest of my life was going to look? I would devour
an entire jar of peanut butter and a box of Ritz crackers in one
sitting, all of it filling my stomach, but none of it filling the
hole in my heart.

Our relationship with food is often rooted in addiction. After all,
addiction is the child of need: the missing parent, a lover's rejection, a
loneliness no heavily booked social calendar can erase. The need to be

accepted and held in safe and caring arms may not be instantly recognizable, but it can be the source of a voracious hunger that demands to be fed. Some handle this better than others. Some are naturally desensitized to the void. Some find creative ways of filling the void. Is it an accident that so many creative people suffer from addiction issues? Not that accountants don't suffer from addiction, nor are they immune to their feelings, but "artists" are often on mental orange alert 24/7. Their feelings are closer to the surface, hence the frequent need to numb the painful ones. It's a twisted web for sure. But what we know is that any form of addiction, be it food, booze, drugs, sex, shopping, gambling, or even just being addicted to feeling bad, comes from a deep place within. So we need to get to the bottom of our needs and wants. Do we really want a second helping of pasta? Or are we habitually trained to shovel some more in to fill that empty space we have been avoiding for so long?

Our ultimate weight losses did not come from dieting alone. They came from a change in lifestyle, a change in attitude, and a deeper understanding of the source of our need. That is not to say any weight plan that limits intake of calories and certain types of food can't or won't work. But if you think you can sustain yourself and stick to a plan that restricts you to carrot juice and kale chips for three weeks, you are not looking at this intelligently. Every time you tell yourself you are on a specific diet or say, "I will never eat another plate of fries," "I promise to give up my mother's meat loaf," or "I swear this is my last bite of pizza," it has the same effect as telling someone not to think about pink elephants. All they'll think about is pink elephants. If you tell yourself you are about to enter the land of permanent deprivation, you will feel despondent and even punished. Your main goal will become ticking off the days until you can return to your old ways. It also opens the door for giant relapses. A bite of pizza can lead directly to three milk shakes, two burrito grandes, topped off with a few cupcakes and a side of chicken wings. (Please pass the ranch dressing.) You may very well lose twenty-one pounds in as many days, then go out and eat your way back to where you were. It's the same exact reason you first identified your issues with the Six Affirmations: Without knowing why you do what you do, no regime will stick and you'll likely be back to your old ways soon enough.

Forty percent of those who lose weight on diets put back not only the lost poundage but additional ones as well. Only a measly 10 percent of those who lose weight on diets actually keep the weight off. This is why we believe diets per se don't work. At least, they never worked for us.

PAUL AND TRACEY

TJ: I did Scarsdale.

PW: I did cocaine.

TJ: I did Jenny Craig.

PW: I did amphetamines.

TJ: I did Atkins . . . three times.

PW: I did Atkins too, with a lot of vodka.

TJ: Any diet where you can have bacon on top of your bacon covered in Russian dressing works for me.

PW: Any diet where I could have vodka in the shower works for me.

TJ: I did pregnant women's urine shots. Lost twenty pounds in two weeks and gained it all back after one tuna fish sandwich.

PW: I did more amphetamines and got a few people pregnant.

However, if you are the kind of person who needs someone telling you what to eat and the exact portion amount, go find the diet that appeals to you: South Beach. North Pole. Food-free. Dairy-free. Whatever. But in the end, if you don't change your behavior and amend your relationship to food, you will not get your situation under permanent control.

Clearly, recovering from a food addiction has problems not faced by the alcoholic or other maxi-indulgers. Abstinence from food would lead to death. You have to eat.

It's worth repeating that one of the most important and workable parts of the recovery movement is the concept of the one-day-at-a-time philosophy. But let's table the food for a minute. We're not here to talk about *what* you eat but rather *why* and *when* you eat. Even though what you eat has real bearing on your weight and health, once you nail the other two, the "what" becomes easier to control.

> "SOMETHING NEEDS TO CHANGE,
> AND IT'S PROBABLY ME."

Of course, to make a change, one needs to know what needs fixing. Time to start digging for the truth. Ask yourself, *What void am I filling with food? Where and when did this start?* Think about what has brought you to this point. Are you gorging yourself to make up for the self-loathing you harbor? Are you starving yourself because you feel that is the only part of your life you can control? Do you stay heavy to keep relationships at bay because you are too frightened of intimacy to let anyone get close? Did you pack on extra pounds when you lost your job? Did you quit smoking and food is the substitute? Do you just lack any self-control?

And why do you want to change now? Is it for the right reasons or a momentary fix? Did someone say something cruel? Did your twenty-fifth high school reunion invitation just arrive? Can't let Kevin Rournik see you with these thirty extra pounds! Did your doctor scare the bejesus out of you? Can you not stand the sight of yourself naked? Do you not want anyone else to see you naked? If we asked you to go take off your clothes and take a long, hard look in the mirror, would you run for the car keys and head to the nearest Denny's? So what makes this time different? Perhaps it's a combination of the above, or, as they say in recovery, you have hit rock bottom?

Mood-to-Food Journal

"SOMETHING NEEDS TO CHANGE, AND IT'S PROBABLY ME."

Any successful business must maintain an accurate inventory of its activities: what's coming in and what's going out. To manage our health properly, we must have the same information. Keeping a daily food journal is not a new concept, but there is no question that recording what you consume on a daily basis—in addition to what you're feeling—is vital to understanding your relationship to food. We call it the Mood-to-

Food Journal. Begin with where you are now and what has brought you to this point. Then keep a record of what you're feeling and what's going on in your life as you make specific food choices. If you can, dig deep and observe the moment-to-moment occurrences around the time you eat. Then keep track of what you eat. This way you can get a handle on your vulnerabilities and how they actively affect the choices you make.

An example: You are at lunch with a friend. You order the grilled fish with a small salad, dressing on the side. She begins regaling you with the tales of her hot weekend in Cancún with her new boyfriend, and before she can get to the second night, you have demolished half the bread basket and are picking away at her fries. This is a far-too-common example of when one starts on the right course and ends up consuming four courses.

Or perhaps you have your wife pack you a healthy, portion-controlled lunch. During a morning meeting you discover the new hire has been given the promotion you thought was yours, and before you can unpack the vegetarian sandwich on seven-grain bread, you find yourself driving through the Golden Arches, yelling, "Supersize me!"

Do you eat ice cream before bed? Do you do it daily? The kids are fighting. Bills are piling up. Do you run for the Oreos? Mood-to-food journaling tracks not only our emotionally triggered behaviors but also our poor daily eating habits—especially for those who might not be overweight but habitually eat foods that are unhealthy.

Something needs to change, and it is probably you. We are not changing you the person—you are swell; we are changing your relationship to food. Your relationship to what you eat and when and why. The goal is to see you develop new lifelong habits that will allow you to find and maintain your ideal weight. Not ours, not your neighbor's, not one of the Real Housewives of New Jersey. By understanding our behavior, we'll be able to keep the present from repeating the past.

"I DON'T KNOW HOW TO DO THIS BUT SOMETHING INSIDE ME DOES."

Clearly on your own you have not been able to tackle your food addiction. It will take more than a set of guidelines from us to completely change such ingrained behavior. That's when you might call on your higher power. If you so choose, invoke him or her and make them a part of your journey.

When you are feeling like you can't do this or you might slip, remember: You are not alone.

Those moments when you know you should get your ass to the gym or your legs out the door and jogging, don't turn to your overused excuses, turn to your higher power and ask for help. As far as we are concerned, the higher power can be your fridge, in which case ask it to hold tight as you try to open the door at three a.m. for that last slice of pie.

> "I WILL LEARN FROM MY MISTAKES
> AND NOT DEFEND THEM."

If you are like most people with a food addiction, your well-worn personal mantra is "It's not my fault." Stop defending yourself to the rest of the world and, more importantly, to yourself. Defending our mistakes is just making excuses—excuses for why we don't exercise and why we can't stick to a diet. In the beginning, we need to be vigilant about observing when we start to defend our behavior. If you hear a defense coming out of your mouth, there is a good chance you are relapsing into old ways. We never have to defend ourselves when we know we are doing the right thing. Think about it: When you order a salad with dressing on the side, or head to the gym at seven a.m., do you apologize for it? Do you say to yourself, *I know I did ten extra minutes on the Exercycle today; I swear I won't do so much tomorrow*? But as that dessert cart rolls around and you take two, do you justify it with *I'm starting a juice cleanse on Monday*? How many juice cleanses have you started and abandoned on day one? Frankly, you don't need to go on a juice cleanse. What you need to do is understand why you compromised your goals for your immediate gratification. What happened? Did you set the bar too high? Did an event occur that took you back to a dark place and to self-soothe you headed for the nearest bakery? Nobody in the real world wants to live on juice. Somewhere between liquefied kale and carb loading is a sensible eating plan. But you need to stop with the excuses.

Take those excuses, write them down, then rip them up one by one.

"I am stressed-out, so I ate." "I found a rubber in Jeffrey's room, so I ate." "I didn't have time to make a healthy meal, so I ordered pizza." "My mother called and started in with the passive-aggressive stuff, so I whipped up a box of Kraft macaroni and cheese and ate the whole thing." The pressure at work, the not having work, all the excuses you return to time and time again to justify why you don't follow through on what you started—these are all problems, but they are not valid excuses. And problems are there to be solved, not made momentarily manageable by eating.

We want you to understand we are not minimizing serious travails and problems. Some of us have more than others. Sometimes they are all heaped upon us at once. Job loss is a horrible situation to be in. The inability to get decent work, support yourself, take care of your family— that is stress at its highest level. With our current economy, boomers caring for their aging parents and often their kids at the same time, fewer decent jobs for college grads, health care still an issue, not to mention broken families, it can feel like the world is caving in on us. It's no wonder depression and mood disorders are at an all-time high. But as hard as it is, please don't use it as an excuse not to take care of yourself. Logically—and we know it's hard to be logical when faced with adversity, impending or existing poverty, loss of lifestyle, serious illnesses that plague us and our loved ones—do you honestly think you will have a better chance of getting a job, finding a new way, or navigating serious health issues if you are tipping the scales to the point of obesity? That's far from the case. You will be much better armed to fight the battles life tosses your way if you have energy, stamina, and good health. If your moods are not ping-ponging from the stratosphere to the dungeon because you overindulged on M&M's, you won't be as easily upset by the daily occurrences we all have to contend with.

Sugar Is a Drug

One of the most common words coupled with *addict* after *drug* and *alcohol* is *sugar*. In fact, there are more people in this country addicted to sugar than to any other substance.

If you think you're just a little overweight but certainly not an addict, take a close look at the amount of sugar you consume every day, including white and brown sugar, high-fructose corn syrup, agave, and honey. It might just dampen your present state of sugar-induced euphoria.

Yes, sugar does indeed cause euphoria. In fact, it tap dances on your brain in many of the same ways that cocaine does. We've all seen kids after a hunk of birthday cake: They're often described as "bouncing off the walls." So while we may not jump around and start throwing pillows, we do get a huge high after a nice, sugary snack. It lingers for a while and then the crash comes: BANG! BOOM! "Holy cream puff, Batman!" . . . and you find yourself plummeting back down to your former state of depression, ennui, sadness, or just plain old blah-dom. So what do you do? You reach for the sweet dopamine rush again. A quick dash to that candy stash will do the trick. Oh, you have a stash? What is the other word often associated with *stash*? Are you starting to see a pattern here?

Sugar makes you feel good. It gives you a sugar "high." Not many other things we eat get the *high* word tagged on to them either. When was the last time you had a zucchini zing, a radish rush, a broccoli buzz?

Sugar is as addictive as a drug too. Since indulging in sugar is not against the criminal code—nobody is going to toss you in jail or take away your kids or driver's license for eating fourteen Krispy Kremes in an afternoon—there is no legal threat to being a sugar consumer and addict. But there are severe consequences in terms of your health and weight.

It's not entirely your fault. While society may snicker at fat people, you can find a shelf of Snickers on every corner. Sugar is everywhere. And many of the foods we eat contain a host of nasty additives that are really just sugar in disguise, which accelerate the addiction process. The manufacturers are not doing their job if you're not coming back for more.

When it comes to kicking sugar, you could go cold turkey, but you might be more successful if you taper it down in bits the same way one detoxes off any other drug. If you are truly obese or overweight, there is a good chance you might be suffering from health problems related to your condition. Before you go on any strict plan, do check with your doctor—although there is no question that it is never too soon to start eliminating sugar.

> ## "I WILL LEARN FROM MY MISTAKES AND NOT DEFEND THEM."

Taking responsibility for our poor choices and not defending them requires understanding and owning the hows, whens, and whys of where we slip up. That's how we set ourselves up for success. If we attempt things that are sure to fail—like crash diets or quitting sugar cold

Enter Except and Accept

I need to lose twenty-five pounds **except** I've tried everything and nothing works.

I would go to the gym **except** I hate to exercise/I can't fit it into my schedule/there isn't one close to my house/who will watch the kids?

I would make dinner myself **except** it's easier to order a pizza than cook. Except. Except. Except.

Time to switch from except to **accept**.

Accept the fact that extra weight is a direct result of your inactivity and overeating.

Accept the fact that carrying extra weight leads to everything from diabetes, to heart disease, and even cancer.

Accept the fact you could be cutting your life short by not accepting responsibility for your own behavior.

Accept that being sedentary seldom leads to becoming slim.

> **"I WILL LEARN FROM MY MISTAKES AND NOT DEFEND THEM."**

turkey—that will only add to our frustration and poor self-esteem, which will send us right back to the cupboard.

Get Moving

Good eating and maintaining a healthy lifestyle are impossible without exercise. Exercise has to be a habit. It has to be daily. It can be varied, but it must be a part of your life.

One of the main excuses people give for not working out is embarrassment. There are many excepts people throw around to get out of this one, but you must accept that you have to just go. You can't be worried about others' opinions—whether they'll think you're fat or look out of place. You can't control what they're thinking, but you can show up. Whether or not you feel fat on the treadmill is irrelevant and temporary, because you are becoming the navigator of your own life.

PAUL

At my heaviest I weighed 187 pounds, almost 60 pounds more than I weigh today. My inflated body and bruised ego dictated my decision to boycott the health club. I didn't enjoy feeling like a stranger in a strange land. I was confused by the machines and lifting less than the girls. Needless to say, I hated it. Getting over it took accepting that what I really hated was myself.

Make exercise a nonnegotiable part of your day; if that means using free weights and an exercise video at home or a Wii Fit, then that is your routine.

   Just remember these three components:

1. It has to be something you like. Just because everyone has jumped on a SoulCycle in the last two months does not mean it's for you.

2. The word *trending* should not be linked to the word exercise.

3. It has to be geographically convenient.

When Comfort Foods Make Us Uncomfortable

It is all right there—*comfort foods*. The English call them puddings or nursery foods. It's macaroni and cheese, mashed potatoes, usually starchy and gooey and warm, often deeply ingrained with Proustian moments. After all, Proust had his madeleine, a childhood treat in France.

   Every country has its version, a one-way ticket back to the early days, a time when we were in the nursery, cared for and quickly comforted, and too often by food. Taste is a powerful sense memory. It's like a warm blanket, a mother's embrace on a carefree day at the beach. It's the temporary reliving of a period when we did not have all these adult problems and issues to contend with.

Who would not want to go back there, especially if all it takes is a plate full of warm chocolate-chip cookies?

Ask most people what their most comforting foods are and they will be able to tell you instantly. They might not know their Social Security number off the top of their heads, but they will be able to vividly recount the exact moment in their life, the people involved, and the precise foods that offered up that comfy, childhood ease.

PAUL

As a kid suffering from migraines, my pain was rewarded with staying home from school, a cold towel on the forehead, and extra-sweet attention from Mom. I was then treated to the traditional "This'll make it better" meal of Campbell's cream of tomato soup and grilled cheese sandwiches.

My mouth just watered as I wrote this. And the memory sent a painful little ping to my heart. It's an eternal sadness that'll always be there. But the combination of tomato soup and grilled cheese sandwiches can still have amazing restorative effects.

There was a time when, faced with a difficult writing assignment or due date I was afraid I couldn't make, I'd take to my bed with a stack of grilled cheese sandwiches. Somehow the work was completed amongst the uneaten crusts, dried Velveeta, and soup-stained cup. Mom always served soup in a coffee cup.

For Andy Warhol, the soup was pop art. For me, it was the love I lost when at thirteen my father was killed in the car

accident and I was shipped off to live with an aunt I didn't
know. I lost both parents, and to this day the symbol of the
safety and love I felt those first few years has been that
special meal.

TRACEY
....

Birthday cake—the cheaper, the better. The more buttery the
buttercream, the happier I am. I have trained myself off sweets
for the most part. I am someone who can have a bite of dessert
and push the rest away. It has taken years, but I can do it,
except in the face of birthday cake. Put one in the room and
you will find me hovering around it. I have been known to
gently nudge small children out of the way so I am first in line.
All I can think about is When will they cut it? How do I
wrangle myself the rose, even though there is only one and
the birthday girl is six and I'm fifty-six? *When no one is*
looking, I take a finger and sweep it across the bottom and take
some icing without leaving too big a dent—and zippo! *I am*
back to being seven years old in front my Mary Poppins cake.
I'm four, with my mom holding a giant Yogi Bear cake in front
of me, my dad next to her. It was a year before they would split.
I can still see my Partridge Family bus cake. I remember a
lemon cake Linus holding his blue icing blanket. A chocolate
troll cake with Day-Glo pink frosting hair. Whatever I was
obsessed with that year got transformed into a cake when my
birthday rolled around.

My mom is cool. She will admit she was more sister and
friend than typical mom. But when it came to birthday parties,

she "mommed" it up. That was when I really was a kid and she
was part June Cleaver and part Martha Stewart, which was
mom enough for me. She threw me well-planned parties with
the cake always being something extravagant. My birthday
parties are some of my greatest childhood memories, and the
cake represents those times. When I am down or needing some
soothing, I usually find myself in a shoe store, but while I
may be soothing with shoes, I am undoubtedly thinking of
birthday cake.

Embrace your past. Own your mistakes, cherish your memories. Understand your comfort foods, your eating triggers, the potholes in your path that cause you to stumble. You don't have to disown them at all. In fact, until you do cozy up to them and acknowledge their participation in your present behavior, they will remain the unconscious motivator and main obstacle in achieving your goals.

"I WILL MAKE RIGHT THE WRONGS
I'VE DONE WHENEVER POSSIBLE."

This affirmation is mostly for those situations where our behavior has hurt or maligned or impinged on another person in some way. For the most part, though, giving in to our food addictions and not caring for ourselves is an assault on us and not others. But one thing it does do is set a poor example for our kids.

If you look at a fat mom, you will more often than not see a fat kid waddling behind her. You might see two. And there's a good chance an overweight dad is parking the car or standing in the popcorn line.

Kids follow by example. If you are eating unhealthfully, they most likely are too. If this is the case in your family, you might want to bring the whole gang on this adventure with you.

Change, especially sudden change, freaks kids out. It also some-times disturbs the ecosystems of the household. When everyone is used to the giant-size soda on the table, the triple-cheese lasagna, followed by the build-your-own sundaes, there will likely be cries of discontent when they are suddenly gone.

It's time for a family dialogue. If the kids are not yet in the danger zone, then explain that Mommy and/or Daddy are changing the way they eat. Talk about the relationship to good health and healthy eating. Tell them you want to be around to play with *their* kids someday. Let them know you are not happy with you and you are fixing it. One of the greatest gifts we can give our kids is the gift of honesty and to teach them how to own their mistakes.

If this becomes a family endeavor, try and make it a fun one. Teach your children that healthy habits can be as enjoyable as the bad ones. Take a family bike ride. Make healthy meals that taste good. Don't stock the house with crap. Make your kids your allies and perhaps your part-ners in this.

> ## "I WILL EXAMINE MY BEHAVIOR ON A DAILY BASIS."

This is not the same as the Mood-to-Food Journal. While the journal is a form of it, this exercise should come at the end of the day after all has gone down. It does not require writing unless you really want to. It is simply taking stock of your entire day. What went well? What could have gone better? Did you set out to exercise and make an excuse and get out of it? Take note of that. Make a plan to not do it the next day. Maybe make up for it by doing a bit extra next time.

On the flip side, did you take the half hour of your lunch break when things were piled on your desk to take a brisk walk? If so, then pat yourself on the back. Do not reward yourself with an Eskimo Pie, reward yourself with knowing you did something that was good for you and on your list.

Were you faced with a crisis? Was it the kind that at one time would have had you running for the nearest Arby's? Did you sit down and write in your journal and have some herbal tea to calm down? If so, you are making progress. Those old triggers are not setting you off the way they once did.

If you gave in to the old impulses, don't beat yourself up; make note of it, instant message your inner Scarlett O'Hara, and have her remind you that tomorrow is another day.

> **"I WILL LIVE MY LIFE IN**
> **LOVE AND SERVICE."**

So you have made some serious headway into the world of change and the achievement of your goals. While you should take some well-deserved time to celebrate your success—hopefully by jogging a few victory laps—the real joy should come from the pride you take in living inside the skin and body of the new you and the fact that you have finally followed through on your promises. While it may sound corny, we think the act of kindness is the glue that holds the new you together. A little bit of love should become your new favorite dessert. But be careful of over-self-congratulatory proclamations; First-person ta-dahs have a tendency to become toxic.

In the world of recovery it's been proven that you get to keep the miracle by giving it away. It is in the service to others that one finds the most rewards. For the alcoholic, that usually means working with other drunks. For the newly recovered food addict, there are other ways to be of service. You might be thinking, *Haven't I done enough here? I have eliminated some of my favorite foods. I'm exercising, journaling, and spending my time making healthy foods. Now you want me to be Mother Teresa too?* Sort of. Kind of. Not really. But the pure energy of doing for others is very real. It's a cosmic currency. And though many will tell you the act of giving is its own reward, we believe there is more to it than that. The returns make service an investment more than a simple act of charity. You will find that what goes out has a magnetic energy that will bring good into your life.

One of the best ways to give back is by starting your own community. Think about heading out in the world armed with your new self-knowledge, your one-day-at-a-time healthy regime, your treasure trove of discoveries made through journaling and daily assessments, and your belief that something out there is bigger than you and that you can rely on it to get you through. Share that with friends and friends of friends and their friends who might need it too. Make a group. Make it fun. Share what you know, talk about how you got there, what happened before, your fears, your triumphs, your setbacks. One finds that as soon as someone has the courage to own what would normally come under the heading of "Shame," everyone else with a similar experience opens up too. And then there is nothing to be ashamed of. You support others in their efforts, and they support you.

You can also start an online community. How many of us love our chat rooms and cyber spots for people who share our interests? So start a health group online. Open the conversation, be brave, and soon you will have many with you. It'll be a great place to go when you feel like you might slip up or be falling back into old ways. It's a wonderful way to share your successes, your worries, and your fears—which you'll most likely have in common with your group mates. Similarly, you can head to our site, www.gratitudeandtrust.com. As many of you may have already discovered, even in its infancy it offers a place to discuss the many issues of concern we blog about there daily. Chances are you'll find potential founding members of your cyber group there.

. . .

A nother way to give back is to focus on taking care of our children. Childhood obesity is at epidemic levels. The schools are still lagging way behind in terms of giving kids proper nutrition and education about how to stay healthy. Many parents just don't know due to lack of education. First Lady Michelle Obama has tried to make this a priority. So why not go into your town and try and help some families that can use the guidance? You can do this through so many outlets: churches, schools, and again online. It's giving the gift of health. It's saving children from lives of bullying, poor health, and setbacks due to the fact they are overweight.

There's power in the word *volunteer*. The energy of caring and the elegance of kindness will serve you again and again in unimagined ways. It's solidly connected to your true goal of living in gratitude and trust.

8.

When You Get to the Fork in the Road, Do You Take the Knife?

How to Turn a History of Bad Choices into a Future of Good Ones

Your Path

1. STOP BLAMING OTHERS.

At this point you might be thinking misfortune always finds you. It's anyone else's fault but yours. But if this is a lifelong pattern, chances are there is a self-sabotager sharing your body with you.

2. DEAL WITH PAST DISAPPOINTMENTS AND LET THEM GO.

For many, disappointment is the only emotion they are comfortable feeling. Look at the ways you have created disappointment and catastrophe in your life.

3. MAKE PEACE WITH YOUR PAST SO IT DOESN'T LIVE IN THE PRESENT.

Learn from your mistakes and don't defend them. Make right your wrongs wherever possible. Then you can start with a clean slate.

4. STOP IMAGINING ALL THE TERRIBLE THINGS THE FUTURE MIGHT HOLD.

Most problems live in the land of tomorrow. Stop yourself when you start a sentence with "If . . ." or "Maybe . . ." Stay in the present.

5. DON'T MAKE MANAGING CHAOS YOUR FAVORITE HOBBY.

Chaos is usually self-generated. Find better ways of feeling connected and alive. If chaos does find you, solve it; don't wallow in it. If you have chaos creators in your immediate family or circle, boundaries are essential.

Does your life tilt toward a long line of poor choices that constantly leave you exactly where you do not want to be? Do you feel like the heavens are shining on everyone and spitting on you? Do you have a history of self-sabotage? When things are finally going well, do you make an irresponsible, poorly thought-out choice that ensures everything falls to pieces? When faced with right and wrong, do you make the sharp turn toward wrong? In other words, when you get to the fork in the road, do you consistently pick up the knife?

Are you guilty of turning your life into something that resembles an Alfred Hitchcock film? Do you regularly plunge a knife into the chest of opportunity? Are you habitually cutting your lifeline to a successful, productive, happy existence? Do you slit the throat of love and passion out of fear?

If so, by now you probably have a PhD in the fine art of screwing up. Your personal history is made up of so many wrong turns, it would leave a gold-medal gymnast dizzy and disoriented. The good news is that there's valuable information in that dented, black-and-blue past of yours.

One of the great truths in life is that nobody gets in our way as often as we do. There are the big roadblocks we put in place and stand solidly behind while positive traffic gets detoured in the other direction. There are the more obvious ones: the food, the gambling, the sex, the booze and drugs. Those are the ones that have more evident physical and psychological manifestations. We get called out on them. People might whisper behind our backs, instigate interventions, or hurl ultimatums: "Stop or else." But there are also more subtle ones that we might casually refer to as our quirks: "You know me; there I go again." But the logical next phase of questions and answers seldom occurs: Why did you go there again? And what choice took you there? Excavation is not so often on our to-do list when it comes to these ingrained life-limiting behaviors. These quirks, issues, peccadilloes, negative character traits, and self-sabotaging ways often get us labeled: "Oh, you know Alicia: Just as things start getting good she finds a way to mess it up." "Wendy, her glass is always empty, but she never seems able to refill it. And if someone tries to do it for her, she dumps it right out." "Frank never has a good thing to say about anyone." "Don't bother trying to please Bob; he will find fault in whatever you do." "If there is a way to screw things up, Cameron will find it." "If there are fourteen nice guys at the party, Janice will find the one jerk." Sound familiar?

Ask yourself a simple question and answer it honestly: *Am I unconsciously creating failure? Am I avoiding success because I don't believe I can handle it or because I don't believe I deserve it?*

What is it about you? What are you actually doing? And where do you go again and again? Are you happy there? If not, then why do you keep returning? What is there that makes you feel at home and comfy despite the fact that it causes pain and gets you no closer to where you want to be? Oh, and one more thing: Where *do* you want to be?

Outside of random acts of bad luck, much of our lives is made up of the sum of our choices. If we choose to find fault, trip ourselves up, and not take advantage of our advantages, then we need to mosey on over to the nearest mirror and yell:

> "SOMETHING NEEDS TO CHANGE,
> AND IT'S PROBABLY ME."

Every day life tosses us endless choices to make, from the mundane to the life altering. *Do I do my laundry or go to a movie?* Nothing profound is going to happen with either one, unless you are down to one pair of clean pants, in which case you should consider doing your laundry first. *Do I marry my high school sweetheart because he's steadfast and asked me, or do I stick it out and wait for Mr. Right?* Anyone who has made a relationship-related decision based on ease and not love will tell you this is the definition of self-sabotage. *Do I stay up late and do a really good job on the report that is due on the boss's desk tomorrow, or do I turn in what I have and go meet up with my friends?* Are you starting to see a trend here? *Do I write that go-screw-yourself e-mail to the guy who is likely to get the promotion, or do I shut my mouth and act like an adult? Do I get gas now or on the way home?* Not an insignificant decision when the tank is blinking empty and you have forty miles to your destination and there are next to no stations on the way home. When you are standing on the side of the road with your thumb out, you have no one to blame but yourself. *Do I call the doctor and get that lump checked out, or do I wait until it goes away on its own?* Need we go on? From merely being forced to wear dirty underwear to possibly jeopardizing your life, there is no end to the ways we humans can sabotage ourselves.

As we have learned thus far, to make those changes, we need to know what actually needs changing. We have tried to isolate some of the top self-inflicted life blocks above, but very few of them exist alone in a vacuum, and one tends to set off a host of others. Poor self-esteem results in self-sabotage; self-sabotage can result in anything from obesity to rage to victimization to treating people badly before they get a shot at you. These behaviors are like a proverbial daisy chain, although they are made up of more thorns than flowers.

The thing all self-saboteurs have in common is they claim to want one thing while their actions lead them in an entirely different direction. Their impulses have a louder voice than their common sense does. They give in when they need to manage, then move past the urge. The same way the drunk learns to not reach for the drink, those who might not be reaching for a drink need to learn to stop reaching for whatever it is that is giving them temporary pleasure (or pain) and keeping them from what they really want and need.

Those who choose the knife over the fork have little or no impulse control. It might be the one trait everyone shares, from the overeater to the serial philanderer to the person with anger management issues. Lack of impulse control is a speedboat ride right up shit creek. So if you want to start traveling in the right direction, you can start by saying to yourself: *SOMETHING NEEDS TO CHANGE, AND IT'S PROBA-BLY ME.*

REACHING FOR A BOTTLE OF DISAPPOINTMENT

Disappointment comes in all types of containers. It's easy to access, as you don't have to go to the store, show ID, or wait until a bar opens. Your disappointment lives right inside of you, and if it's not there, you can whip it up faster than the Iron Chef can chop a carrot. You know the recipe: Add one part past history to a few heaping cups of fear—a pinch of anger and resentment are optional—blended with the most important ingredient: the feeling that nothing will ever turn out the way you want it to, so you might as well disappoint yourself before someone else can. There is a good chance Disappointment was the diet of your youth. You grew up on it. It's the meal you run to as opposed to digging into a healthy dish of Maybe This Time Things Will Work Because I Deserve to Be Happy.

Just because the past is littered with discontent, though, does not mean the future has to be.

But for many, that disenchantment is the devil they know. And while it's heartbreaking and self-defeating, we reach for it time and time again. It may not propel us into a drug-induced stupor, but it can cause us to feel that the deck has been, and will always be, stacked against us. That feeling of futility then sends us to the mall to max out the Visa and MasterCards. Or it might lead us to bed to indulge in a three-way with

Ben and Jerry. It can hurl us into a dark vortex of pain, the result of which is many forms of negative behavior. As destructive as it may be, this way of responding to life is sought out and nurtured because it is the emotion we are most familiar with.

Do you delete your dreams as quickly as they appear? Do you find fault with others before they can find fault with you? Do you look at a possibility, a person, a situation, and instantly toss it into the "Never Going to Happen" file? You might not even be aware you're doing it. It's a reflex, turning your back on the challenge of success and retreating to the familiar landscape of defeat.

Reaching for a bottle of disappointment often grows out of our childhood experiences. If yours was a childhood tainted by cruelty or unhappiness, the sense memory of that repeated behavior lingers into adulthood and leaves behind a quiet fear that nestles deep in your unconscious. Early introduction to anxiety leads to an apprehension about life that can be hard to shake. The stress of that always-expected random attack keeps a fight-or-flight response continually floating on the surface or just below.

The thing about reaching for disappointment before disappointment reaches you is that you always remain in control. There will be no surprises. No way, no how, is anyone going to hurt you. You will put a kibosh on that before they have a chance. The disappointment "reachers" have a leg up—or so they think. For us, nothing beats knowing the negative outcome, not even the chance of a good outcome. And as much as we hope, pray, conjure, and fantasize another way to be in the world, the satisfying job, the healthy relationship, the "This time it's working out" feeling is dwarfed by the sense of "I would rather know where I stand than take the chance of being disappointed again."

While living on a bottle of disappointment will not demolish your liver or get you a mug shot, it can and does have its own damaging effects. It can thwart you from making choices—any choices. It can keep you stuck in neutral forever in order to avoid the chances of a possible disappointment ahead. But by downing our own self-generated bottles of disappointment and making sure nobody slips us a Mickey, we not only maintain a misguided sense of control, but we also tend to remain in a constant state of depression.

Reaching for disappointment isn't always idling in the same place; it can be active. Reaching for a bottle of disappointment can take the form of always making the wrong choices, such as picking the wrong mate. It's ending up with the same person even though they may have different names, jobs, backgrounds, and hair color. They are the same person in different form, whether it's a lover or a friend. But they all share one trait: They are sure to let you down. They will on some level be unable to deliver what you need, want, desire, deserve. There's the codependent, the married man, the ice princess, the taken, the narcissist, the sadist, the masochist—pick your "-ist." For it's no fault of yours that they are damaged, right? But whatever it is, it is sure to not work out. The operative word there being *sure* . . .

TRACEY

If there is one addiction that has plagued me for much of my life, I would have to say it's reaching for a bottle of disappointment.

I was the girl who always picked the wrong guy. Even if he wasn't the wrong guy for someone else, he was the wrong one for me. I was going to change him and make him right. Of course that is impossible. It only took me until

I was forty and had been through one bad marriage to figure that out.

There is no question that much of it goes back to my father, who left when I was young and has been out of my life more than in it. He is also one of those people who for no reason is suddenly mad and not speaking to you. That made me hyperalert. I was always trying to figure out where I stood with people. I would take the blame for things that were not my fault.

If Daddy can't love you, then there must be something super-wrong with you. Right?

It's not that I didn't envision happiness, love, or reliability; it's just that I didn't understand how to sustain it. And there was no question that I feared what would happen if I got and then lost it. I didn't know how I would get through that again. So better to be in a situation I knew was doomed from the start. I also always had fifty reasons why I didn't really like someone in the event they dumped me.

It was a terrible way to go through life. I ended many a friendship because I did not want someone hurting me first. It took a lot of therapy and really owning that the responsibility lies with me. I could no longer blame my father for my poor choices. If I wanted to be happy, I would have to take control. It only took thirty years. Hey, better at midlife than never!

Reaching for a bottle of disappointment is booze for the control freaks. Booze makes you happy, then takes you down. Then you take more and the cycle goes on. It numbs the pain until it wears off and the pain doubles with guilt and the preexisting condition. But in reaching for a bottle of disappointment, we know what we are getting, we know where we will wake up and with whom. There are few surprises. It all stays the same—sucky. And we know sucky. And it's all going to be sucky anyway. So let's just stick with sucky.

So the next time you catch yourself sidling up to the disappointment bar for another round, stop yourself and say: SOMETHING NEEDS TO CHANGE, AND IT'S PROBABLY ME.

And let the process begin.

Stuffing Is Only Good on Thanksgiving

Are your true feelings stuffed into the bottom of your emotions drawer? Are they hidden there for no one to find? Do you swallow words and thoughts because you're afraid if you own them you might be judged, shunned, abandoned, or ridiculed, or you'll have to actually deal with them?

Where is that closet where you've crammed every hurt you didn't mention, every abuse you didn't acknowledge, the betrayals you let slide? Is that closet filled with so much crap it looks like an outtake from *Hoarders*?

Are you worried that if you try to open the door to expunge them, they'll fall on your head and bury you? If so, consider the alternative. Stuffed away, these things will start to meld into one big uncontrollable emotion called resentment & rage. And from time to time we're willing to allow all that R & R to pop out and land in the lap of the wrong recipient.

Misplaced anger and rage are very common when we don't deal

with them in the moment or with the right person. So your kid gets the whammy you've been holding against your mom for years. Your boss gets the lacerating e-mail you wanted to send your neighbor who ran off with your wife. Your dad loved your sister more, so you find yourself taking it out on your best friend.

Feeling avoidance is at the root of many addictions and maladaptive behaviors. But feelings do not disappear just because we wish them away or stuff them down. They come back in oh so many ways that wreak havoc on our lives and relationships. If any of this rings a bell, it's time for some emotional housecleaning and a resentment purge.

Feelings can be scary, especially those we have already ascribed the role of Bogeyman. Assigning the right emotions to the correct situations and people is the best place to start. The affirmations done properly will take you there.

"I WILL LEARN FROM MY MISTAKES AND NOT DEFEND THEM" and "I WILL MAKE RIGHT THE WRONGS I'VE DONE WHEREVER POSSIBLE" are essential for getting to the core of your sealed-away emotions. There is great healing when you can go to your child and say, "I'm not angry with you; I'm upset at things that happened with Grandma. I am sorry for whatever hurt I've caused you." You then need to go to Grandma and deal with whatever you have spent your life avoiding.

It's about living authentically, giving our true feelings the space and attention they deserve. Dealing with issues in real time, before they have time to fester and grow, saves an enormous amount of pain and indignation. Once you have a tidy emotional closet, you will never want to see it messy again.

THE IFS AND THE MAYBES
OF IT ALL

All ifs belong to the future, and even then, they don't necessarily live there. More often than not, they are dangling somewhere in the land of make-believe. But they take root in our fears and then grow into scenarios that feel more real than reality.

Many ifs have a negative connotation attached. *If* I lose my job, what will I do? This is a valid question to ponder, especially in this economy. And one does need to make adequate preparations (if they can) for the possibility of a rainy day. But there is a big difference in acknowledging that a rainy day could be in the future and walking around with an umbrella perpetually perched above your head.

PAUL

My wife, Mariana, has a whiplash-you-back-to-reality saying that's an effective antidote to needless worry: "Two ifs and a maybe."

When she catches herself, myself, or a friend worrying needlessly over some imagined catastrophe that might happen in the future, she chimes in with "Two ifs and a maybe."

Stop and think about that one for a second. How many

*of us zero-to-sixty ourselves into high anxiety based on an
imagined notion of what could happen down the line?*

*We do it with everything: our health, our jobs, our families,
our finances—you name it. We can two-ifs-and-a-maybe
ourselves right into disaster. "If my boss hates the report and if
he likes the new guy's better, then maybe I will get fired." "If I
did lose my wallet and did not just leave it at home (where it
likely is) and if the people who stole it take all my credit cards
and max them out and take all the money out of my ATM,
maybe the bank won't reimburse me and I will be deeply in
debt with no funds."*

*One of the most common two ifs and a maybe occurs with
health: "If this pimple is in fact a tumor and if they don't catch
it in time, I may be dead by Christmas."*

Stop me now. I can go on all day.

*The lesson being when you find yourself starting a sentence
with the word* if *and you hear a* maybe *creeping up in the rear,
stop yourself and make a vow to worry about any of this only if
it actually happens, which it likely won't.*

These ifs and maybes are the double-edged knife for the self-
saboteur. It might not sound like self-sabotage, but it can be one of the
worst kinds. If your ifs are not totally catastrophic, then at best they are
drawing all your attention to the future and nixing your ability to fo
cus on the present. When you are residing in a future state, you are not
living in the present and thus are not engaged and centered. You are
worrying about what could come to pass as opposed to dealing with,
accepting, and being grateful for what is occurring in the moment.

We set up false future scenarios that justify the destructive choices in our lives. "I will be happy if I lose the weight." "Maybe once I meet the right guy, I will get my shit together." "If my mother would stop controlling me, I could maybe move out, find a job, and take charge of my life." "If my boss were not such an asshole, I could do my job better." "Maybe if my wife had more sex with me, I could lay off the porn."

These are all conditions. And they are predicated on other people's behavior. As we know, other people are responsible for their behavior, and yes, maybe your boss is an asshole. But what does that have to do with you and your performance? You do the best you can. You might get another job out of it. Your boss may see value in you that he never has before. Or he may still be an asshole because he is one, but you need to derive pleasure from your acts, your accomplishments, your knowing you are playing your A game, regardless of other people's personality disorders.

One can see the shared characteristics between the substance abuser and their loved ones with the if-and-maybe people. "If . . ." and "Maybe . . ." are used as excuses for not leaving, not invoking tough love, and not setting boundaries. These all being forms of codependent behavior.

"If I tell him to stop drinking, he may leave me. He may find someone who lets him. He may hurt me. I may not be in control." It goes on and on. But again, it is living in a future state and not reality. No matter what the if or the maybe, the outcome is never a good one.

A day at a time is the way it goes in recovery. That allows for living in the moment. There is no "*If* I have another drink, *maybe* just this once . . ." The ifs and maybes are removed as they imply conditions over which we have no control. And that does not allow for responsible, grown-up actions.

TRACEY
....

I'm not in recovery but I have been in therapy for many
decades. And I can't see leaving anytime soon. Just when I
think I am free to go, my therapist says something that is so
revelatory I realize I could be a lifer.

Recently I was talking about various people in my life and
sharing some events—nothing earth-shattering; it all veered
more into the realm of annoying more than anything. But he
said, "You are treating all these people 'as if . . .'"

He continued, "From everything you have told me, this is
in keeping with who they are. This is the way they always
behave. Why do you treat them as if they were someone else?"
People are continually let down by others because of the
inability to accept them for who they are and then treat them
accordingly. It's much easier to "as if . . ."

Taking the knife is handling a difficult situation with "I will just
treat you *as if* you don't have this problem, because then maybe it
will go away." This is a total setup for disaster. "You're not a narcissistic,
self-loathing, angry, disconnected, verbally abusive, physically abusive,
anorexic, controlling, out-of-control, remote, reckless, hoarding, frightened, sadistic, masochistic person. If I don't address this directly or treat
you or myself as if this is going on, well, then maybe it isn't." We avoid
what we are frightened of. If-ing is a great way to avoid.

There is no end to the dysfunctional behavior we attempt to deal
with "as if" it weren't there. We even treat ourselves this way. Nobody
gets over anything by being treated "as if" they already have. In fact it
often just intensifies the situation. Why would someone actually face

something and amend it if those around them already behave as if they have? They are already being rewarded for work they are yet to do. Where is the motivation in that?

TRACEY

We had a crazy dog called Melvin. Melvin was cute but had more than a few screws loose. He used to do this thing where he would get all wacky and start to shake. His eyes would glaze over and usually the next thing that would happen is he would pee. Wherever this attack happened to take place, he would just haul off and piss.

For some reason his favorite place to flip out was our bed. I used to take the attitude of "Pretend it's not happening; just ignore him." If I pretend he isn't wigging out and it's all okay, then maybe he will forget about it. Of course, this never worked, and he would pee all over our bed. Usually right before we were about to get in it.

Many a night was spent washing sheets and drying the comforter with a blow-dryer. Eventually we had to give Melvin away. Had we dealt with his "condition" early on, might we have been able to help him and thus keep him? I don't know. Melvin might have been one of those beings who enter your life and you have to let go of.

But one thing that I know didn't work was pretending he was okay.

Granted, it's not always easy to fix the broken parts. And we accept that certain addictions are illnesses. But if you treated someone with heart disease "as if" they didn't have it, they wouldn't be given the opportunity to get well. One of the biggest problems with diabetics is the fact they often live "as if" they did not have the disease—and it ends up doing them in.

Look at your life—how many places do you find yourself "as-if-ing"? How much of your own maladaptive behavior and that of those around you are you pretending does not exist and therefore not dealing with it properly?

The smaller things can be let go of. Oftentimes there are things that—if we merely see them for what they are and stop attempting to "as-if" them into something else—we can learn to live with. We can let go of unrealistic expectations, which only lead to unhappiness. We can stop thinking we are going to please the malcontent, be it our parent, boss, child, friend, or coworker. People who don't like themselves find it impossible to really ever like anyone or anything for very long. We don't need to assume someone who has never responded the way we wanted or hoped will now respond as if they were someone else with very different traits. You can't treat the irresponsible as if they were dependable and then be disappointed when they behave exactly as they always have. You are not accountable for their poor characteristics, but you are responsible for seeing them for who they are and not "as-if-ing" them into another type of person.

Then there are the bigger deals, maybe even the deal breakers— the ones we really don't want to face head-on, as they would require a lot of work to fix or perhaps serious emendations to our lives. It's easier to "as-if" them into submission.

But the real lesson in "as-if-ing" is that it only makes things worse. It often cements us to our problems and them to us. It prevents us from moving forward and finding the bliss in healthy, honest living. "As-if-ing" perpetuates the myth that all is okay.

We don't necessarily stop loving people when we acknowledge their flaws. The same goes for ourselves. In fact, it is actually the opposite: Love comes from acceptance. And sometimes it means we have to take the big step and trust that by not "as-if-ing" anymore, our future will be healthier and thus happier than our past.

Living in the Land of Chaos

Do you know anyone whose life is in a constant state of chaos? Do controversy, drama, and blow-ups seem to be a part of all their interactions and relationships? Does a cyclone of dizzying energy enter the room with them? Of course you know people like this. We all do. Some of us might even be them, the souls who have chosen chaos as their home address. They are addicted to drama, pandemonium, confusion, bedlam, turmoil, and disorder. They feel comfortable only in commotion. They feel in control when everything around them is in disarray and madness reigns.

They find it easier to yell than to talk calmly. They prefer to blame others than to take responsibility. They constantly change their minds but often forget to change their clothes.

They endlessly sabotage themselves, their relationships, their jobs, and their chances. But they also leave those who come in contact with them confounded, depressed, worried, and many times wondering if they are in fact the ones who are crazy.

Who are these people?

They can be and are everyone, like the roommate who comes home every night full of complaints that morph into verbal attacks, which suddenly have the whole house nervous and all attention focused on the perpetrator, his moods and erratic—though predictable—behavior setting the tone for that evening and sadly often most evenings and days to come.

It can be the boss whose tumultuous hysteria puts the whole office on edge yet oddly makes him look like the calm captain steering his ship through rocky seas.

It can be the moody, self-involved, angry teen who, no matter how much you do for them, turns every event, conversation, question, and outing into a test of who can scream the loudest.

They can be schoolteachers, ministers of finance, truck drivers, mothers, heads of state, and presidents of movie studios. They're everywhere. And while they're self-sabotaging in many ways, they are often high-functioning in others.

PAUL

There's a very famous Hollywood producer who became known for constantly creating chaotic environments where only he and he alone could function. Thrive, in fact. The orderly world around him would be intentionally destroyed and thrown into a state of disarray. His coworkers and competitors alike collapsed under the weight of their own confusion and cracked egos, while our egomaniacal producer, empowered by his sense of control, would emerge a leader.

Control. Was this his ultimate goal? Was there a sadistic pleasure in the destructive episode, somehow reminiscent of the

bully on the beach kicking sand and knocking down the other
children's sand castles? Why would anyone behave in such a
horrific fashion?

While the creators of calamity come in all ages, genders, and socio-economic groups, the one thing they often share outside their love of life in the emotional wind tunnel is that they somehow all end up being victims of other people's actions. They over-salt the soup, then complain about the meal and blame someone else for wrecking it. They react hysterically, using out-of-control responses as a defense: *"Why are you doing this to me?"*

So where does that leave you? Often those who are surrounded by chaotic people have a difficult time interpreting what is real and what is not. They wonder what part of this mess is their fault—and if, perhaps, the buck should have stopped somewhere else and not in front of them.

Children who are raised in chaotic households either become chaos seekers themselves or they wind up as emotional Sherpas carting around the heavy bundles of other people's misplaced emotions. People who live in the land of chaos either do not want to leave it or they don't know how. So some sit with their articles of discontent as the only things on their radar, wailing behind a curtain of victimhood, while others try and talk sense to people who, for all intents and purposes, will never hear it. Or they crank up their own volume until screaming becomes the language of the relationship. Attack, retreat, defend, yell—all with nothing ever being solved. The thing it does manage to do, however, is keep most interactions high-octane and often contentious.

For those who live with or come into proximity with these drama kings and queens, it is a very unsettling experience. Why would people constantly make things so hard for themselves and those around them? Like many forms of maladaptive behavior, it's addictive. There is a certain endorphin rush involved for some. They find tumultuous but familiar thrills in simply surviving at the center of the storm. They are very squeaky wheels and they get a boatload of grease. For some people, it is the only way they know how to exist. Chaos is their form of communication; it's their way of life.

If you've recognized chaos as either your permanent location or fortress of choice and you've arrived at a place where you are tired of living your life in a continuous typhoon, then say it with us:

> "SOMETHING NEEDS TO CHANGE,
> AND IT'S PROBABLY ME."

It will cost you too much in the long run to continue along the catastrophic highway.

> "I DON'T KNOW HOW TO DO THIS
> BUT SOMETHING INSIDE ME DOES."

Be patient, you didn't become this way in a day; it's a process. But hopefully you will look back at some point and wonder how you survived your own self-created storms or the storms you put up with in others.

> **"I WILL LEARN FROM MY MISTAKES AND NOT DEFEND THEM."**

This affirmation is key to changing your behavior. Justification is a weapon for you, and you mustn't reach for it out of habit. When you find yourself explaining away the wreckage of your past, remember these words and regard them as a flashing red stop sign. An emphatic denial or excuse can undo any good you've accomplished with your new behavior.

> **"I WILL MAKE RIGHT THE WRONGS I'VE DONE WHEREVER POSSIBLE."**

Take your time with this affirmation. There will be many opportunities to rescue friendships and repair the damage done. Be patient with yourself and those around you. In the world of recovery "More will be revealed" is a promise of unimagined healings.

> ....
>
> ## "I WILL EXAMINE MY BEHAVIOR
> ## ON A DAILY BASIS."
>
> ....

If you're the one wreaking havoc, clearly a history of creating chaos will leave a trail of damaged relationships and a history you would love to rewrite. Your journey now becomes one of self-discovery and corrective engagement with the world around you. The extensive list of wrongs you must right will diminish quickly if you make the Fifth Affirmation a nightly habit.

For those of you who live with or must deal with chaos-seekers, you too must change. It's easy enough saying, "It's not my problem." As we have seen, and as you know, you'll only end up on constant hurricane watch, often meeting the other person at their level of hysteria. It's not always easy, but it's up to you to alter the language of the relationship, especially if you are dealing with someone who is not going to change themselves. Many will not, so the proverbial ball falls in your court. The most important thing you can do is change how you respond.

Chaos likes to deal with chaos. If you keep your temperature down and don't try and argue sense with someone who is making none, you will find yourself in a position of control. It doesn't mean you have to be the dartboard while they toss them at you; it means stay steady and stay focused on the information and not the hysteria. It also means sometimes it's best to walk away. Don't do so in a huff, as this will only throw fuel on their already rapidly accelerating fire. Just walk out of the situation calmly and say, "We will revisit this when you calm down."

Granted, these are Band-Aids, and all Band-Aids eventually lose their adhesive, but it does accomplish one important thing: You are no longer embroiling yourself in someone else's ongoing hysteria. And you are not making yourself frenzied in the process.

There will always be people who choose the knife over the fork, but hopefully after years of self-"stabotaging" many will eventually pick the healthier route.

9.

Navigating the Nasties

*The World Is Full of Imperfect People
and You Can't Avoid Them, So Let's
Learn How to Deal with Them*

Your Path

1. THE WORLD IS FULL OF UNENLIGHTENED NASTIES: YOU HAVE
TO ACCEPT THEM.

But accepting their unappealing character traits does not mean you
have to respond in kind. Take stock of the jerks in your life and figure
out what category they fall into, detachable or attached, then figure
out how to deal with them.

2. YOU CAN'T TEACH AN OLD DOPE NEW TRICKS.

Don't preach. Don't cajole. Don't fall back into old patterns. Nothing is
quite as unnerving and liable to send you back to former states of
maladaptive behavior than a tyrant pushing your buttons. And they will
try. Especially when they are faced with the newfound calm and
centered you. If the going gets tough, get going. That could mean
walking away from a dinner table, quietly hanging up the phone, or
packing your bags. The story and your part in it will dictate what
action to take, but don't try to get them to see the light or expect them
to be influenced by you. If anything, they may become threatened and
try and provoke you into action. If the language of the relationship has
always been combative, then that is what the aggressor knows and
feels comfortable with.

3. IF THEY WON'T CHANGE, YOU HAVE TO.

Most people will not change until they are good and ready. And that
may never happen. So you will have to invoke your iron will and
repeat your mantra: *Something needs to change, and it's probably me.*

We know you have changed, but what you must do now is change how you deal with the nasty personalities in your life.

4. YOUR PAST CHOICES DON'T HAVE TO BE YOUR PRESENT REALITY.

Many of us have made choices based on our tarnished pasts. If Dad was a nasty piece of work, there is a very good chance that guy snoring next to you might share many of the same traits. Now that you are on the road to becoming healthy, you have to decide how to deal with the people in your present who are holdovers from your past. It's harder when we are bound by legal ties and offspring, but there are ways to break free.

You are starting to really like that person in the mirror. Not just physically but the inside as well. You have replaced excuses with acceptance, and you are taking responsibility for your part in mistakes and misadventures. You have made amends to those you might have dinged, dented, or damaged. You now catch yourself midding or sometimes pre-ding and make corrections in the moment before real damage can occur. You end each day with a pat on the back and a positive plan for improving the next one. Old habits you thought would never die have not only begun to disappear, but most of the time you actually don't know where to find them. Positive behavioral responses you had to work hard at incorporating now come easily and are often your first reaction. Smiles and thank-yous have taken the place of gripes and *if only*s. You're rocking.

Most people seem to have noticed your transformation, and maybe have congratulated you on it or expressed their appreciation. But then there's those people who, no matter what, still give you a hard time. What's wrong with them?

NEWS FLASH: The world is filled with nasty people and we have to learn to live with them.

It is sadly the truth. You can overtip the waiter and he might still growl at you. You can bend over backwards to try and make your cranky, judgmental mother-in-law happy, but she will still find fault with everything, from the way you load the dishwasher to the way you parallel park. There will always be those for whom you are never good enough because they themselves don't feel good enough. There will be others who are jealous of your progress, and again, there are those who are just plain nasty. Often born that way. Sometimes bred to be such, the intersection of nature and nurture still being one of the world's great mysteries. And then, of course, there is anger, resentment, jealousy, laziness, addiction, and all sorts of other issues we have discussed that lead people down the path of jerkdom.

No behavioral change on anyone's part is likely to affect them. Until they come to the place where they can utter, "Something needs to change, and it's probably me," they will likely remain recalcitrant, angry, bitter, controlling, critical, nitpicky, and just plain difficult to get along with.

We are married to them, work for them, live next door to them. They are our kid's friend's parents, our oldest pal from high school, our drunk uncle, our narcissistic roommate, the guy at the gas station who snarls when you pull up. Your banker, postman, or third cousin twice removed. They're people we merely bump into or are tightly tied to as we scroll through our lives. Nastiness knows no politics, crosses all socioeconomic borders, and is not gender-specific. It is just part of life. And thus we need to learn how to deal with it.

Oddly, when we were playing the blame game and not owning our own crap, others did not seem to smell as bad. But as one cleans house, all of a sudden the neighbor's trash becomes more obvious and annoying. So how to deal with these nasty characters becomes a bigger issue.

While compassion, caring, and forgiveness are the preferred tools to use in order to keep us lovingly connected to the world around us, the butterflies-and-rainbows lifestyle is tough to maintain when face-to-face with a full-tilt, card-carrying asshole. Accept the fact that the days of your life will include face-to-face encounters with these seemingly unfeeling, unenlightened idiots.

The question then becomes: What to do when forced to interact with a grown-up bully who may have been a cactus in his last life? In the recovering community there's a wonderful expression: "God made the assholes too!" The point being that there's a reason tucked away in the most unpleasant cretin's past that probably guided him to his current dead-eyed state of nasty. Understanding the cause may make the symptom—the behavior you're suffering from—a little more tolerable.

The thing about dealing with jerks is that each case is different. How you handle them depends on several factors. First, there's the toxicity factor. How bad are these people for you? Do you walk away from every encounter with a particular person feeling like hell? Do they have a way of saying the most banal thing that instantly turns your mood from Gandhi to Himmler? Do you walk into a room full of confidence and on contact with said aggressor suddenly doubt everything from your nail polish to your second child's name? If so, "Whoops, time to go!" may be the exit line that's safest and most effective, although it is not always possible. Your tactics will depend on what role in your life that particular person plays. We've found that the nasties can be divided into two categories: detachable and attached. Simply put, there are some people in our lives we can shake more easily than others.

Detachable

These are people to whom we are not attached. It could be the casual friendship that has run its course and now only leaves you feeling wrung out and kicked in the teeth. Or it could be a significant other. You may say, "But my boyfriend and I have been living together since high school and are now in our thirties; how much more attached can you get?" You are not attached. You are merely in a situation you have not taken the steps to extricate yourself from.

You might be attached by property, finances, promises made, papers signed, early dreams commingled, but those are just details. They might be hurdles, but hurdles are meant to be cleared. They are not reason enough to keep you living in a state of constant agitation or regret. Your future should not be dependent on threadbare details from your past.

We all know when a relationship is not good for us. It may take us time to own it and actually verbalize it, but once you do that, once you declare a relationship is causing more pain and frustration than pleasure, it's time to seriously think of leaving. If you're hiding keys or money, fighting, leaving and returning, crying yourself to sleep, lighting candles in hopes that things will change, repeating mantras that things will change, or standing on your head in the hopes of gaining a clearer perspective, then your present situation is not working. Have your friends and family been hearing the same stories about your not-so-better half for years? Is "I would leave except I don't want to lose the apartment/lose the dog/be alone/have to look for a job/pack up/divide the books and furniture/move in with Mom/go to back to grad school/ cut back on my standard of living/sign up for Match.com" your defensive position?

You might be attached by financial strings and shared interests, and it might be too costly to break those immediately, but there are gentle ways to sever ties and seek a healthier life. But first you have to really accept where you are and stop making exceptions.

TRACEY

There was a point during my first marriage when it was clear I was desperately unhappy. I found endless ways to avoid dealing with these feelings directly. One of them was remodeling the house. I had a theory that as long as we were working on the house, our union was somehow healthy and moving forward. People would ask how we were and I would say. "Great. We are doing over the den." Nothing could have been further from the truth. We were not great at all, and I was terrified that we were quickly running out of rooms.

At one point I went to a therapist to talk over my feelings about my marital situation. For the first year I talked about everything but. I think I spent a lot of time complaining about contractors.

I remember getting in the car after every session, driving down Santa Monica Boulevard, and thinking two things. The

first one was Whew—you got through another round without
saying a word. *And the second one was* You need to come
clean about this. You are wasting your time and money. But
if you actually own the problem, it won't be a secret anymore,
and you are going to have to fix it. *It was something I was not
willing or wanting to do at that point. Lying felt safer.*

*Eventually I changed therapists: I found a smarter one who
saw through my façade and by the second session said, "Let's
talk about what's wrong with your marriage." Busted. It took
many years to walk away, but the long march on the road of
truth had begun. I could no longer lie to myself about myself.*

So what do you do? Sometimes silently—or loudly—leaving these
people in your past might be the best way to go. Silently is sometimes
the easiest and cleanest—although there is something cathartic about
gently letting someone know where their behavior could use improving.
The fact is you probably aren't going to change their conduct on the
spot, but if you respond to rudeness with a noncombative, quiet reflec-
tion of what it feels like to be treated in that fashion, you might have a
positive effect down the line.

To quote the late, great lyricist Hal David, "If you see me walking
down the street / And I start to cry each time we meet / Walk on by . . ."
This is a profoundly healthy way to play it. We need to recognize that
we are crying—not because of something we did, but because of the
way someone treats us. And then we have to find the strength within us
to *walk on by.*

We are tethered to people in so many ways we seldom understand.
And the unhealthier the relationship, often the deeper the unconscious

activity we are trying to fix or extricate ourselves from. Walk on by. So much easier said than done. How many times have we walked on by and gone sprinting back as soon as the opportunity arose? It frequently takes more strength to keep going than it does to hang out in a familiar yet painful situation.

This is where *Something needs to change, and it's probably me* comes in very handy. Sometimes, changing means moving on. It means knowing the other person is not going to change; therefore you have no choice but to be the one who takes control and walks away. Change often means changing the situation you are in by removing yourself from it.

Since your partner, friend, or lover is not willing to face the reality of the situation, the fact that you are leaves you in the position of power. Heavy is the head that holds the knowledge, but powerful is the person who knows what he or she has to do to make their life a calmer, more productive, happier place.

As the writer Paulo Coelho says, "Close some doors. Not because of pride, incapacity, or arrogance, but simply because they no longer lead anywhere."

Do it as gracefully as you can. Hurt as few as possible. But accept that anytime others are involved, people will be hurt. They will recover, though; time and distance do heal. Someone has to be brave. Someone has to declare, "This is not working. If it's not working for me, it can't be working for you." Someone has to carry on and move. The situation has to change, and it's you who is going to change it.

The nasties can change and many do. But if they aren't in the process of doing it now or moving toward doing it anytime soon, you might need to cut them off.

TRACEY
....

The years have taught me that in every dysfunctional, unhappy relationship there is usually—almost always—one person who finally gets up the guts to end it.

In one of the unhappiest, unhealthiest relationships in my life, I was the one to say, "No, this cannot go on." It took a long time. I kept going back. If I had not walked, I might still be there, wringing my hands in anxiety and sharing the state of my misery with all who would listen.

I am an observer of people and their lives. I most always hear from my friends or those who share their stories with me: "It was I who left. He/she would still be there had I not moved out/on." Many people are perfectly willing and are often content to live lives of quiet or screeching desperation. It's what they know. Moving on, saying good-bye, closing one chapter and starting a new one takes bravery, courage, and an acknowledgment that things are not working out and they never will. It requires that bold first acceptance that something needs to change, and to admit to oneself: Since the other person in this duo is not about to do the changing, it's going to have to be me.

Attached

But what about those individuals who are permanently attached? Of course, some of the nastiest we are forced to deal with are those we can't just walk away from. They remain in our lives—and our faces—

for what feels like and often winds up being eternity. One out of two marriages ends in divorce. If you happen to fall into that minuscule, marginal 50 percent of the population, there is an excellent chance your ex could be a jackass. If you were not fruitful and did not multiply, it is much easier to leave your unhappy past where it belongs. But if you do share offspring, you are unfortunately, for all the right reasons, stuck with your ex-nasty, who is in fact more than likely still a nasty. In which case you have no choice but to learn to deal with this soul in a healthy way that does not cause all your internal demons to enter the room or, worse, send you back to your old unhealthy habits.

What to do with the bullies and tyrants that happen to be attached? How do we muddle through this without engaging at their level? The first thing to try would be *I don't know how to do this but something inside me does*: Turn it all over to whatever higher power you might be relying on. Mind you, this does not always work. But it does have a way of kick-starting your compassion. Once compassion is in the driver's seat, you are not as likely to throw a flowerpot at your ex-mate the next time they come by to pick up the kids. What you might be able to do is see their damage for what it is. Acknowledge they are the way they are because of a multitude of components that were in place long before you entered the picture—and, as you can see from your present vantage point, have not diminished one iota since you exited it.

Once you have cleaned up your side of the street and vigilantly kept it swept, other people's problems are not your fault. Many of us are codependents and blame everything from the situation in the Middle East to our partner's porn addiction to some character defect in ourselves. As you have seen by invoking *Something needs to change, and it's probably me*, culpability is king. But culpability is not possible for everyone. Just because *you* do it does not mean your posse or ex-posse will follow.

So if you have a powerful inner Mother Teresa, compassion may pull you through. You might just be one of the few who can look at the damaged and the uncontrolled manics/maniacs and take pity on them. Give them some tea and sympathy. You might be adept at turning the other cheek. It's an extremely rare gift. If it weren't, those who have it would not usually end up with *Saint* before their name.

There are times when we can mutter "Poor them" to ourselves. Acknowledge it's not our fault, then smile, nod, pretend we are listening, and agree while we are secretly balancing our checkbooks in our heads. We can then close the door, breathe a sigh of gratitude that they are no longer playing a costarring role in the story of our lives, and return to those relationships that are healthy and sustaining. Or just sit down and binge watch the entire first season of *Breaking Bad* and leave these unfortunate beings behind. Though that's not always an easy path to take.

We want to yell, "You moron, don't you realize the pain/drama/ heartache/headaches/destruction you are causing?" The inclination to whip out a laundry list of their faults and a how-to guide to fixing them is so appealing that we find ourselves biting our tongues to the point of bleeding. But as we have learned, it seldom does any good for those who are not capable of hearing. So bite we do. Smile we do. Bleed we might. It's one way of dealing with an impossible person we are forced to encounter on a regular basis and are unable to walk away from. And of course there are the people who are incapable of walking away, no matter how untenable the situation may be.

Without question, the trickiest tyrants to extricate ourselves from are those we are related to. There is not a person alive who does not have some relative—distant or immediate—who is not a certified member of the Nasty Party. Obviously when they are your third cousin seven times removed, it makes walking away or nodding hello and then making a dash for the deviled eggs at a holiday gathering easy. But what about those of us with jerk parents or siblings?

Sticking around in miserable relationships is one of the most common causes for anxiety, depression, and sometimes even addiction. A loveless, abusive, or absentee parent is more often than not the root cause of many of our codependent and bad choices.

We often seek what we know. If we know a parental figure to be a problem and we have not worked it out, we will more often than not go and find their clone and start the whole game over again, this time with the mantra *I am going to make it right*. If our parents let us down due to their own character defects, you can bet at some point we will head out into the world and try and attempt to rewrite history.

Did Daddy drink? If so, there is likely to be a drunk in your future. You couldn't fix Daddy, but this time . . . just watch! (How well does that one work?) Was Mommy depressed and distant? Let's go hook up with an unattainable ice queen and melt her into an emotional, warm love bunny. (Not so fast . . .)

Not all parents with character defects are nasty. *Nasty* is a pretty strong label. It is reserved for someone who hurts others without awareness and apology. Who is downright mean, abusive, self-centered, and destructive. These people are the parental Terminators, a breed all their own. Anyone who has been the offspring of one can tell you in vivid detail the traumas they wrought.

PAUL
....

Having been the jerk on more than one occasion, this is
a troubling issue for me. My "picker" was broken for years.

*I picked people to share my life who were simply the wrong
fit. In the beginning of those relationships, the friction heated
things up in a passionate fashion, probably born of unconscious
needs—on my part and on my partner's.*

*A few years on the analyst's couch threw some much-
needed light on the subject. Unconscious desires to write new
endings to old stories played a large part in my past choices.
Being sent away as a child created abandonment issues
that often drove my psyche into dead-end territory. Likewise,
meeting a woman whose dad was a drunk and missing in
action made me the perfect choice to prove history didn't have
to repeat itself.*

*Wrong. The same dynamics led to the same results. So, as
a recovering jerk, I look at current creeps I encounter as sick.*

*It's the single most effective choice I've been offered in
processing resentments. There will always be people who move
through my life and yours whose every word will affect us like
fingernails on a blackboard. You can grind your teeth and
mumble insults to the jerk du jour or you can take that deep
breath and try the one thing most likely to do any good: Pray
for the son of a bitch.*

So the question constantly crops up: What to do with the impossible parent? We wish we had a one-size-fits-all response. How willing
and able are you to leave behind those who gave you life? Some can do
it with ease, while others will take almost any crumb of attention simply
to maintain some contact.

"Walking on by" and abandoning parents is less difficult when they
are alert and vital than when they start to get older and infirm: Stories

of deathbed reunions between estranged children and parents are legend. Few wish to cross over to the other side with unfinished family business left behind. And then, of course, the guilt for those who remain can haunt them until they too are on their way out.

If you fall into the first group, hopefully you have made peace with your decision and don't carry any resentment with you. We are sometimes masterful at saying we don't care. Yet underneath the bravura lies a hurt, needy child who spends his or her life looking for Mom or Dad in all the wrong places. So if you walk on by, be sure it's what you want to do and try and do it with as little rancor as possible.

If you are going to stick around and have made internal peace with the fact that Mom or Dad flunked the Ward and June Cleaver School of Parenting, be sure you have boundaries in place. Boundaries are huge, especially with parents. And one of the biggest complaints you hear from those with disrespectful, disruptive, disappointing parental figures is that they have no boundaries whatsoever.

Minding your personal family business may be cute in the land of sitcoms, but in the real world such meddling can be terminally destructive. Establishing boundaries requires a firm and unyielding stand against what may seem an unstoppable force. The maternal tsunami of disapproval may unleash a flood of emotional havoc that turns your psyche into a montage of bad memories and makes sleepless nights the norm. The child of anxiety is more anxiety. But you are an adult now; you can speak up. Nobody is going to send you to your room or take away your favorite doll. So setting clear lines indicating what is okay and what is not is perfectly acceptable and recommended behavior. No need to keep swallowing your feelings only to get a stomachache from so much impacted hurt and frustration. Remember, there is nothing wrong with gently pointing out cruel and uncalled-for behavior.

"It hurts me when you call me a slothful bitch" is something that needs to be verbalized. How the other person perceives it is not your responsibility.

Physical boundaries for the abusive are to be considered as well. Keeping yourself and your family protected from those who are not safe is not only advisable but required. Immediate departure from a physically abusive encounter is the only sensible move. When the house is on fire, get out first, then call the fire department.

That said, one person's distance is another's person's prison: It is so situational and dependent on personality. You have to find what works for you. Some people can repel manipulation, whereas others are sucked into its vortex. It is important when dealing with family members to identify their behavior and your go-to response. If you start to feel your buttons being pushed and the old response about to erupt, try to make an adjustment. Know this is old, habitual behavior that you can now change. It can be as easy as saying, "I am going out to get some air." Then you can quickly call upon your higher power: *I don't know how to do this but something inside me does.*

The low-hanging fruit of family tormentors is often our siblings. They say no two children are raised exactly the same way despite the fact that they share parents. This is because they don't have the same siblings. Siblings can be the cause of some of our biggest issues, family fights, jealousies, perceived inadequacies—the feeling that we can never measure up. They can also be a source of great strength and companionship through life. But let's go with the ones who phone in as nasty.

Much like with parents and ex-spouses, there is an incontrovertible lifetime connection, but there are many siblings who opt out of a close or convivial relationship. If you happen to be one of those people burdened with a difficult, unwilling-to-change sibling, you pretty much have the same choices you do with the other intimidators in your life. In fact, siblings are easier to ignore than parents. They can sometimes be placed in the category of "Friends We No Longer Have Space For." We can talk to them when we have to at family events—although there are many who won't show up at family functions if the loathsome sister and her orangutan husband will be in attendance. But these are all the quotidian life details you have to navigate on your own.

Many of these situations that you once found intolerable can be turned around by employing the Six Affirmations. Since these individuals are not going to change, you can change your attitude toward them. Where you once might have shot back with a rapier retort upon your brother digging at you for the four thousandth time about something that happened six years ago, you can smile and say, "Good to see you, Brian," and walk on by. Seek out some other life-affirming relative. Not responding totally disarms. But many of us have been so locked into dysfunctional family dynamics for so long that we don't know any other way than to respond. There was a time when you would have zinged one back to Brian and reminded him of some long-ago misdeed or maybe asked him if he had found a job yet. Didn't the unemployment run out two years ago? Before long you are deeply embroiled in the same fight you have been having since you were four.

Now something has changed: It's not Brian, it's you. Brian cannot push your buttons anymore. He has only the power you give him. So you don't have to rob yourself or your family of time together because some of the people you happen to share DNA with are Neanderthals.

Let's take this to the next level. Maybe Brian has a way to get to you like no other. Out of his own misguided habits, he sees you and goes for the jugular. And perhaps this is not the best day for you to have your cage rattled by your obnoxious brother. You find yourself swelling up with those old feelings and the aggression that is the language of your relationship. You know the expressway to Brian's Achilles' heel better than anyone, but that does not mean you have to take it. In this case, walk on by. Take a breath. Do it. Just take a breath. When in doubt, try to channel your inner Gandhi, breathe, and change the topic. If you cannot muster the detachment to do that, then extricate yourself from the situation. Go find a quiet place and draw on your higher power: *I don't know how to deal with Brian but something inside me does.* Maybe you don't need to leave; maybe you can stand in front of Brian and silently say: *I don't know how to deal with Brian but something inside me does.* Wait a moment. Find something neutral to say. Then go help yourself to some of Mom's deviled eggs.

What happens if Brian is so enmeshed in this dynamic he can't leave well enough alone? Maybe he is threatened by your newfound calm. WTF happened? You guys have been battling since you were in diapers, and now you've turned all Hare Krishna on him. But Brian knows you well, so he sidles up to the buffet table, refuses to let it go, and brings up some long-ago affront on your part. Brian may have no self-awareness, but he has extraordinary long-term memory, especially where your mistakes are concerned. So he nails you with one. Smirking. *Let's see you karma chameleon your way out of this one*, his smile says. But unbeknownst to Brian, you are prepared.

You don't yell, you don't scream, you don't jam a turkey carver in his groin; you just quietly say, "You know, Brian, I made a lot of mistakes during my life, and that one in particular taught me [fill in the blank]. Our mistakes can be amazing teachers. No one makes deviled eggs like Mom."

Brian has a lot of unresolved issues, none of which he will own. He can hold a grudge longer than David Blaine can hold his breath. Siblings being siblings, humans being human, you have undoubtedly hurt his feelings. Maybe in your "wrong righting" you left out some things. When one is making amends, things do slip by. But ol' Brian holds on to it like a teddy bear. The familiarity of your encounters has comforted Brian for decades. It's the place he can run to when he remembers he's a screwup. It allows to him to relive hurts you dished out to him. He relies on you being as cruel and unfeeling as he is. That way he is not alone. So, mouth full of deviled egg, he reminds you of the hideous, hurtful thing you did back when *Ghostbusters* was the number one movie in the country.

He's waiting, he's chewing, he needs you to lash out, he wants that same ol' feeling you two have shared your entire lives. He *needs* the anger. He lives off the hurt. Something needs to change, and it has not been Brian. But it has been you. And so maybe you say, "Wow, Brian, I forgot about that. I am so sorry. I have done some really unkind things in my day. And that must have really hurt you. I wish we had talked about this sooner. But let me apologize now. My intent was never to hurt you. I was dealing with my own stuff. Or not dealing, as that event points out. Sorry, bud."

If Brian chokes on the deviled egg, your impulse might be to walk on by. We are only human here, after all. But instead, offer him the Heimlich maneuver. Your seismic shift has taken him to places he was not prepared to go. Brian knows only one way to interact with you, and by your changing your position, you have totally altered the dynamics of the relationship.

As you lay your tryptophan-overloaded body into bed that night, you can mentally go over your exchange with Brian. You can be proud that you did not revert back to your old ways. Thanksgivings do not have to end with you and Brian doing your version of mud wrestling with the leftover gravy on the kitchen floor. You can take the higher road. It's not always easy, but telling people off, pointing out their faults, and re-creating past patterns of negativity—as we have learned—get us nowhere on the path to a better us.

You might even say a little prayer for Brian in whatever way you pray or speak to your higher power. Maybe you can ask your HP if he/she/it can help Brian not be such a jerk. It has to be hurting his life. Or maybe you just nod off in gratitude that you are not carrying around the anger, quick temper, and grudges that are clearly weighing your brother down.

All that said, if the whole family Thanksgiving vibe is too much to deal with and the amount of energy you'd have to put out to deflect all the negativity would sap the Thanks out of the day, you might want to volunteer at a soup kitchen next year. At least that would cover your love and service part.

Take the Garage Door Opener Away

I used to facilitate group therapy for the Musicians Assistance Program. A sober musician I was working with constantly complained that his younger brother kept pushing his guilt button about not being there for him. There'd been no dad present in their home and he'd been the only father figure.

> He wasn't going to drink over it, but the repeated nagging was ruin-
> ing their relationship. One day I asked him if he owned a garage door
> opener. He did. I wondered what he'd do if his little brother kept open-
> ing and shutting his garage door. "I'd take it away from him," he replied.
> I suggested he metaphorically do the same thing now: deny him access
> to those buttons. If the musician would stop responding to the jabs, even-
> tually his brother would get bored and stop. The quarreling about the
> past had become the language of their relationship, and for the younger
> brother it was proof that he wasn't alone.
>
> By refusing to participate in the old dialogue, the two began to con-
> nect around other, more constructive elements, both played music, and
> their relationship grew. Happily, once a jerk doesn't mean always a jerk!
>
> —Paul

There is yet another type of attached asshole. While not attached by blood or previous history, they are attached by necessity. This would be the workplace asshole.

Everyone has had to deal with the boss/coworker/team member who wears his meanness on his sleeve. As we observed in Chapter Eight, blowing up these relationships will do you absolutely no good. The "I don't deserve this; you can take your job and stick it up your butt" e-mail you stay up all night writing in your head will only get you tossed out on yours. And letters of recommendation are not likely to be com-ing your way once you have pulled that trigger.

So what are your options? No one wants to be miserable all day, but work is work. It's not your love life. Being unhappy because your coworker is insecure and belligerent and takes all the credit is different from living with someone who through their passive-aggressive attacks leaves you feeling like roadkill.

Work, by its very nature, is a competitive and often combative environment. Lovely is the image of the utopian workplace where everyone has each other's back, benevolent bosses treat all equally, and there's free full-time day care. But that's so far from reality that it barely exists on TV anymore. So we must be accepting of the fact that work will be trying. We will be forced to deal with jerks on a regular basis. In fact, the workplace can also bring out the sweetest guy's inner bully.

Don't misread this and think we are saying, "Tough luck." What we're saying is that, in the same way you employed the affirmations with a difficult family member, you can and should do the same to get through your daily interactions with the people you are forced to deal with at work.

If you take the time to understand that all people who act aggressively, cruelly, or underhandedly are deeply insecure, it might make it easier to sit through those morning meetings without wanting to stand up and tell them off once and for all. Something needs to change, and it's obviously them, but your telling them that will not help the situation at all.

You might want to knock on the door of your higher power too. *I don't know how to deal with this schmuck, but something inside me does.* If you go to that place, some amazing answers may make themselves known.

Or perhaps, much in the way you disarmed Brian, you just don't let it bother you. We can't control how other people behave toward us, but we can always control how we behave toward them.

We are all animals; it is our nature. When attacked, animals tend to attack back. Fight or flight is part of our survival technique. Chances are the old you fought back when you were feeling attacked. It's hard not to. But while we may be animals, we are people too. So step back. Disengage. You do not have to defend yourself. You now know how to learn from your mistakes and you don't defend them. Do your work, keep to yourself, interact as much as you have to, and do it on a strictly professional basis. You don't need to make everyone your friend. Not everyone is going to like you, especially if you have something they want or they perceive you as a threat. Just because the workplace tends to be dog eat dog does not mean you have to bite. In fact, you might stand out if you refrain. But you don't have to be a doormat either.

If someone is outwardly unkind to you or a defenseless coworker, a quiet, sincere description of how you feel when he or she assaults you is more productive than attacking them back. Exchanging the pronoun *you* for *I* takes the onus off of them. Even if they are the responsible party, "I feel . . ." always keeps the sensitive feelings with you and leaves little room for a counterattack.

The nasty boss might be the hardest one to deal with. Authority figures, especially those who write the checks we live on, have a powerful place in our lives. They not only by their very position have the ability to control us, they also conjure up all sorts of emotional sense memories that stem from our parental units. The transference of boss to father/mother figure is a common one, be they benevolent or maniacal.

It is much harder to set boundaries with your boss unless he is sexually abusive. If he's just a run-of-the-mill nasty, you're stuck with him—unless you want to quit and find another job. This is when your affirmations come in handy. Keep your side of the street clean. Do your work. Do not do anything that can get you in trouble. Bad-mouthing him behind his back may feel good, but that can be used against you.

Plus we are now hopefully beyond resorting to those tactics. We all hate to be underappreciated, verbally abused, made to feel inferior, taken advantage of. But you are not a victim here, so playing the part of one only feeds into your past behavioral patterns. Much like with a diet, you can choose not to eat the cake. The consequences are not worth the momentary pleasure. Take the same stance with your boss. You can leave if you want to, but you choose to stay. The consequences of leaving a paying job are too high. So you trundle forward, trusting there will be days when you won't know how to do this but something inside you will. You understand that something needed to change, and it was you. Your boss needs to change too, but chances are he won't. So act and don't react. Learn from your mistakes and don't defend them. Own when you are wrong and be confident in your abilities when you know you have done the right thing. Make right your wrongs wherever possible. Continue to examine your behavior, and if you see it edging toward a place you won't be proud of, pull back. And, as always, have gratitude and trust. Be grateful you have a job. Unless you are a trust fund baby or sold your start-up at the right time, chances are you need one. When the going gets rough, get googling and see the unemployment numbers. That alone should make you grateful you have a paycheck coming in on a regular basis, even if Captain Curmudgeon is signing it. In fact, knowing that might make him look a little better to you.

Work is tricky. It's called work and not play for a reason. It's supposed to have *hard* before it and not *easy*. It's what we do to get by. So we don't get to pick who is in charge and who is not—unless of course we are lucky enough to be in charge, in which case go to the Fifth Affirmation right now and examine your behavior. Are you a nasty boss? If the answer is yes, then something needs to change, and it's you.

10.

The Ones We Love

I'm OK, You're Not: How to Help Those Who Don't Know How to Help Themselves

Your Path

1. USE YOUR NEW LIFE TOOLS TO HELP YOU DEAL WITH THE ADDICTS IN YOUR LIFE.

Most of us know someone, are related to someone, or are exposed to someone who is addicted to a substance. Are you making excuses for someone? Stop. Is your "helping hand" actually destructive enabling? Stop. Are you preventing someone from hitting bottom, which will scare them into finally changing? It's time to stop.

2. CHANCES ARE, WHATEVER YOU'VE BEEN DOING HASN'T WORKED.

Once you have exhausted the usual paths—intervention, pleading, threatening—it's time to let go. The addict is powerless over the substance and you're powerless over the addict. You can't do the work for them.

3. THREE IS NOT ALWAYS THE CHARM.

Rehab and intervention don't always work the first few times. Be prepared for relapses. Your addict could get clean on the first try, or it might take years. You must stay centered and not relapse into your old enabling ways. Take care of yourself. Remain optimistic: You never know what the future holds.

While we're focusing on the life-limiting habits and addictions many of us suffer from, we'd be remiss if we didn't discuss the people in our lives who might need help doing the same. It's difficult to find a human being who is not connected in some way to a substance abuser. It can be someone as distant as your barber's brother's wife's cousin or as close as the life partner sitting across from you.

Family and friends are usually trained to cover for the offending alcoholic or drug user and pretend there is no serious issue. Cars parked half on the driveway and half on the lawn are quickly moved before the neighbors can see them. Spouses too hungover to go to work can count on their mates—no matter how upset—to pick up the phone to cover for them. "Steve has a touch of the flu and won't be in today. I know this is the third time this month." In households around the world, that scenario is played out again and again. The income is too essential, the truth too humiliating, the façade too important to ever let the truth slip out. It's a dangerous lie to keep living, but one people cling to—often for decades.

It's not just family that gets this special "The issue is safe with me" treatment. Far too frequently friends and coworkers take on the burdensome role of keeper of the secret. It's often done in the name of love, but in truth it's only aiding and abetting. And it makes for a relationship filled with resentment, embarrassment, and sometimes rage.

Is there a best friend you often need to take the car keys from after a girls' night out? A child whose Halloween photo from the year he dressed up like Spider-Man adorns your mantel who now imagines real spiders crawling up his arm when he's in the throes of drug-fueled hallucination? Spouse, friend, child, neighbor—most people know and care for someone who's involved in the deadly dance of untreated alcoholism and addiction. If it is a close family member, it has all the makings of a living nightmare.

And how you love to share the details of those hours of agony with your addicted child, husband, brother, or friend! How could they put you through such pain? You point your finger and state the facts of life as seen through your suffering eyes. In most cases the fighting, pleading, or blaming becomes the language of the relationship. Sadly, the buck stops with you in this situation, as unless you alter *your* behavior, this will continue to be the controlling dynamic of your bond even if the party stops using and abusing.

While the first affirmation, "Something needs to change, and it's probably me," may seem an inappropriate tool to reach for when you are clearly not the problem, it will prove an effective stance and offer much-needed relief. "But wait," you protest. *"I'm* not the addict here. *I'm* not the sloppy drunk who keeps dragging this family through revolving-door dramas again and again. Why would *I* need to change?" Here's why: The energy expended in a repetitive, high-voltage game of tug-of-war with an addict will leave you drained. The cost of living your life fully invested in the recovery of an addict unwilling to change is much too high.

So how can you exist in the quiet comfort of gratitude and trust if your loved one is an addict? How do you stay balanced, productive, and sane when your child is hopelessly addicted to drugs or your husband has a permanent seat at the neighborhood bar? The phone ringing late at night stops your heart because you're afraid it's the police or hospital calling with news of some narcotics-induced disaster. You live that moment in your mind again and again, suffering the dark fantasies of a parent whose child or partner is playing chemical Russian roulette.

First, understand that you are not dealing with issues of character flaws or moral misbehavior. Yes, your alcoholic partner or offspring may be acting out in a myriad of unacceptable fashions while under the influence of his drug of choice. But they're actually sick. Their ability to make rational or even moral choices is greatly diminished under the influence of a chemical dependency. It's the only explanation for why your Honor Roll freshman daughter or Eagle Scout son is suddenly pilfering cash from your purse or selling household items to pay for their habit.

You are dealing with the side effects of a chronic and potentially fatal medical condition. That fact was proven by the Jellinek study, and alcoholism was recognized by the American Medical Association as a disease more than fifty years ago. Your addicted relative or friend isn't some spineless miscreant unwilling to use a little willpower to lick this thing. Once they're under the influence of their drug of choice, the ability to hear the sensibility of your arguments is minimal. Escaping the clutches of addiction is a monumental task. Trying to talk an addict in need of his drug into choosing abstinence is like trying to tell a hungry lion that too much meat is bad for his cholesterol.

The roller coaster rides of hope and disappointment are eternally frustrating, not to mention scary. Living with an addict you love means living in perpetual fear. Fear leaves us feeling hopeless. Hopeless means in the absolute we have lost control, and in the case of the addict, you *never have* control. Whatever substance is in play has firm hold of the steering wheel.

Begin by arming yourself with information about addiction. You'll discover that many of the actions you've taken again and again in an effort to help have hurt your addict's chances of getting sober.

Addicts in need are possessed by their cravings. Quitting usually requires more than just manning up and saying no. To safely transition, they will need close supervision and very possibly a medical detox. It's a myth that people die from heroin withdrawal and not from alcohol withdrawal. In fact, it may be more common the other way around. The nervous system reacts violently to the complete removal of alcohol after long-term consumption, and seizures may occur without transitional medication of some sort. Detox needs to be medically supervised. And rehab is a powerful asset in learning how to live clean and sober.

Because you have tried and failed does not mean you should totally throw in the towel—not yet at least. There are some ways of dealing with the addict that do work. It depends on the nature of the addiction, the personality of the addict, and oftentimes how long the addiction has been going on.

Intervention

In the last thirty years, intervention has proven to be a powerful tool in getting an addict or alcoholic into treatment. Statistics suggest that there is virtually no difference in the percentages of success between those addicts who choose to enter treatment on their own and those who were confronted with an intervention. The impact of family members gathered together as a group to inform the patient that help is available can be a powerful ally.

PAUL

I spent a few days at a clinic that offered instruction in intervention techniques. I've been an active participant in a half dozen cases. It's an interesting process that has a kind of "improvisational theater" energy to it. You prepare family and friends for a surprise meeting with the patient, usually a family member who's slowly killing him- or herself with alcohol or some other drug. The unsuspecting addict is then confronted with a calm and civilized collective expression of concern and love. At least, that's the planned route to reclaiming their life.

The idea is to gather the tribe around the subject of the

*intervention and quietly share their personal stories of how
the addict's being intoxicated around the clock has made life
unnecessarily complicated. The message from each member
of the intervention team is "We can't go on living with your
current behavior." Examples are given of the horrors of life
with———, and after gritty and detailed illustrations of the
client's past behavior are shared, the "gift of life" is offered.
The suitcase is already packed, and a car is waiting to whisk
them away to treatment. Arrangements have been made in
advance, and all that's left is for the patient to say, "Yes, I'll
go. Thank you. I knew this was coming; of course you're right.
It's time to get the help I need."*

    *In my limited experience, this sort of friendly persuasion
doesn't always happen as planned. A sobbing wife screaming
at the top of her lungs and referring to her mister as "a sloppy-
ass drunken son of a bitch who's out of my life for good if you
don't get your shit together" is not uncommon. "I'd rather be
dead than go to rehab!" is sometimes the last thing you hear
before the client walks and the door slams. Sadly, that self-
fulfilling prophecy is sometimes the end result. Still,
intervention remains a sensible option.*

In a perfect world, the result of an intervention is as planned. A
suitable rehabilitation site has been chosen and the patient agrees to
commit to whatever program is deemed appropriate for their long-term
recovery. Life begins again as all enter into a period of newly learned
behavior.

    But do not lose hope if your addict refuses at first; they might sur-
prise you in the weeks ahead. Many times the person who refuses treat-

ment at the time of confrontation will come around later. They may not. They may try and fail. It may take three or four trips to rehab before it takes. It's a rocky road to rehabilitation, so tighten your seat belt. You are likely in for a bumpy ride.

Boundaries

Hopefully the gift of life you offer your loved one will be accepted, joyfully or begrudgingly, and will lead to a sober lifestyle. It may not happen. And if he or she agrees to go to rehab, it may not be enough. You may hock your wedding ring to get Junior fixed, and he may repay you with a celebratory bender as soon as he clears the doors at Betty Ford.

That's why boundaries become key when dealing with the wet drunk or using drug addict. While your strongest instincts may be to jump in and "fix" the log-jammed life of your loved one, by saving the day you will do more harm than good. Paying rent, phone bills, lawyers' fees, and traffic citations, and dealing with the endless parade of economic calamities created by irrational behavior, allows the identified patient to continue on his or her unhappy way. A road that often leads to insanity or death.

Obviously the rules are very different when dealing with an underage child. You are legally, physically, and morally responsible as a parent, and as such, you have the right to inject discipline at a level greater than with someone of legal age. You can place his or her misbehaving little butt in rehab and sign away your life savings to keep them alive and get them healthy. You do everything you can. It's what a good parent does. But addiction is cunning, baffling, and powerful. What to do when the teenage years have slipped away and in their wake you're left with a young adult who bears little resemblance to the sweet child you remember?

Consequences

Consequences are often key for an intervention to succeed. If the addict can refuse help and return to life as he or she knows it, they will promise anything to do so. "Give me a few days to clean things up at the office." "Now? The holidays are coming. I'll go in January." "I have finals. I promise when the semester is over." These and all other arguments need to be ignored. You might have put your foot down before. But how many times did you pick it back up? Addicts are stellar at playing to one's sympathies. They are often some of the most charming people you will meet—at least until the substance kicks in and turns smooth-talking Jekyll into chair-throwing Hyde. So charm they will. Cajole until you are weak-kneed, broken down, and longing to believe that this time is it; you will go along with most any lie or solution they propose. But if your methods of "fixing it" haven't worked in the past, they won't start working now.

Consequencing anyone we love or care about is very difficult to do. Remember your parents right before a spanking (back in the days before spanking was close to a felony): "This hurts me as much as it hurts you"? And you're thinking, *Right. I'm the one with the blistered butt.* There is truth in it. When one throws down the proverbial gauntlet, there is a lot of fear attached. The big one being: *If I make this demand of them, they are likely not to love me.* If we remember that anyone living for an extended period of time with a drunk or addict is in a codependent relationship of some sort, chances are they have their own issues to work out. Most healthy people—really healthy people: the kind that are hard to find—have one or two repeated negative encounters with addicts and they take a hike. It's much like women who are abused. There is a type of woman who will be hit once and that is it. She is gone. Then there are the ones who stick around. It might be time for you to go.

PAUL

I've stood more than once at the end of that pointed finger, responding with calm reasoning or angry accusation. In my disease I had one specific goal: Let nothing separate me from my drugs. My medicine. And to that end I mastered the high art of denial and fabrication. I became an expert at lying through my teeth.

After a brief period of abstinence, I started using again on a trip to Jamaica. I returned to the States and soon to my full-fledged addiction as well. My live-in girlfriend recognized the change and very lovingly called me on it. "You're using again, aren't you? Let's get you some help." My response was immediate and heated—what I now see as sadistic. "What's the matter with you? You have a lot of issues with men, don't you? Something inside you is broken. What did your father do to you?"

The tirade continued until, in the end, she'd go upstairs to bed, alone and in tears, doubting herself and wondering if there was, in fact, some truth to my accusations.

There was none. And there was nothing wrong with her perception or her instincts. I chose my drugs over her and her feelings. No matter the cost. Addicts can be powerful, convincing, and sometimes heartless in their fight to avoid

change. In the end she left me. I now see that as a gift. It was
what I needed at last: someone willing to dump me if I was
unwilling to change.

Using the Affirmations

So what can you do? How can you help someone who doesn't want
help? How can you reason with someone whose only reason for being is
to get to the next fix or drink? You've paid for interventionists, footed the
bill for rehab, and pleaded. Pleaded until you couldn't stand the sound
of your own voice. But all efforts have failed.

> **"SOMETHING NEEDS TO CHANGE,**
> **AND IT'S PROBABLY ME."**

As hard as it is, for your sake and in the interest of those around you,
your behavior needs to change. You need to stop trying to control the
alcoholic. Whether the identified patient throws in the towel and sur-
renders to the process or continues to use for years, you need to recognize your own codependent participation in the ongoing dysfunction
and adjust accordingly.

There are things in life we cannot fix, no matter how much energy
we may devote to them—no matter how badly we may hope, desire, and
dream the situation will just get better on its own. That kind of magical

thinking never plays out in the real world. This is the instance where you have to hand that power over to something outside yourself. It's the first move the drunk takes when he vows to get sober. You must follow suit, even if you are the first to make the move. You need to change your mind-set and realize that, just as the alcoholic is powerless over alcohol, you are powerless over the alcoholic. Sometimes nothing is the best thing you can do.

> **"I DON'T KNOW HOW TO DO THIS BUT SOMETHING INSIDE ME DOES."**

How, then, can you shift your thinking based on a number, eighteen or twenty-one, and close shop on the "Mom and Pop to the rescue" reality show you've been participating in for years? It's hard. But for you as well as the addict, there is freedom in surrender. You are incapable of changing someone who isn't ready to change. Quit. Give up. Your goal is to release. It's time to pursue the art of letting go. Take comfort in the knowledge that you are no longer in charge. The truth is you never were.

By not pushing, pulling, yelling, and demanding, you are not giving up: In fact, it's the opposite. You are taking control over your part in the ongoing drama by merely stepping back. You are allowing a process to take over that relieves you of the hopeless task of trying to influence something you have no ability to change.

Oddly enough, the best options you have may seem heartless and uncaring. The list of things you might try are almost all counterintuitive to your normal parenting, loving ways, or laundry list of Judeo-Christian good deeds. If the addict is a danger to him- or herself or others, calling the police may be necessary. A thirty-six-hour forced psych evaluation may be called for. Not an easy thing to do to someone you love, but you may save their life in the process.

You're changing the rules, and the rewritten facts of life need to be communicated. That family member who's been turning to you again and again to save the day needs to know that there is no longer a lifeguard on duty. It may require changing locks on doors and refusing to accept collect calls, but the rules have to be adjusted and it won't be welcome news.

Often you have to walk away—hard to do when you have been hanging on to the addict's dysfunction like it was a life raft that would keep you both afloat. If they don't go, which they seldom will, you must. If they refuse to go into treatment, you need to remove yourself lovingly from the situation until they do.

If the addict is unwilling to accept help, your choices are few. You must allow him or her to hit bottom. You will hear this again and again from those who hit it and those who had to stand by helplessly and watch. There is no feeling more agonizing than watching someone you love dearly give their life to addiction.

> "I DON'T KNOW HOW TO DO THIS
> BUT SOMETHING INSIDE ME DOES."

Reaffirming your own spiritual connection is a must once you have changed the rules. Having come to that impasse where walking away was the only thing that would work, you may have lost contact with your problem child, husband, or sibling. It's time to realize that all of us are on our own path with our own higher power. That immense power is there when we are willing to reach for it.

When those late-night nightmares of your son or daughter being homeless and broken interrupt your sleep, you will need to strengthen your own belief in that inner ally. Know that energy or supreme being is available to everyone. In the world of recovery it's described as "turning it over," which you will have to do again and again. Give the care and feeding of your errant offspring to the universe and know that you are doing the best you can by simply praying for guidance and the highest good of all concerned.

There is hope for the hopeless. But only they have the power to commit themselves to a clean and sober lifestyle where rehabilitation and the continuous act of recovery becomes the most important thing in their lives. People all over the world get sober each day. At this very moment, 10 percent of Americans are living in the world of recovery.

New beginnings are strongly flavored by wishful thinking for the co-addict. A few days of abstinence offer such promise and hope. If your addict awakens to a sober morning and returns to you clear-eyed and committed to recovery, rejoice. But be cautious. Trust is earned, of course, and time will tell the tale. Remember that this is a life-long process. Remind yourself that you are no longer the keeper of the keys. Monitoring the daily comings and goings of another, watching for signs of harmful behavior, can become a head-spinning routine that will eat up your own days and nights. You cannot live in that constant state of agitation and worry.

Thus, often you have to leave them to do what they will and step way back.

If they are successful in maintaining a sober lifestyle, celebrate with them. Be as supportive as possible and let the relationship grow in trust with time. Keep in mind that abstinence alone is not recovery. Recovery is a lifelong commitment. It's a choice. It requires honesty, patience, and vigilance. It's a lifestyle and it's a lifesaver.

TRACEY

If someone you love needs help, there are abundant resources available. Among the best are those wonderful organizations listed at the front of the phone book: Alcoholics Anonymous and Al-Anon. They will work with you if you are willing to work with them. For both the alcoholic and the codependent, they offer specific programs that have saved lives for decades.

11.

Gratitude and Trust

*The Cornerstones of a Happy,
Centered Life*

Your Path

1. RECOGNIZE YOUR SUCCESS.

Give thanks for the positive changes you've made. Take a moment to honor what you've done. A quiet celebration is in order, and not just in this moment but each day and often. As we become grateful for the world around us, we become grateful for the world within. When we are grateful, there is little room for negativity or fear.

2. PASS IT ON.

The essence of living in gratitude and trust requires giving back. Make your search for ways to be of service a part of your daily ritual. "Lead me where you need me" is a powerful request; say it often. And when the answer appears, follow.

3. STAY GRATEFUL.

The nature of life's journey includes potholes, bumps, and bruises. Survive with dignity and humor. Avoid the panic of the abandoned; ignore the urge to return to well-known but destructive patterns. Trust that you are being cared for and be grateful for all that comes your way; there are lessons in the imperfections, light in the darkest places. Make it your habit to always find it.

Repeated use of the Six Affirmations, combined with the appropriate constructive action, will lead us to an emancipation. With the chains of old habits and destructive behaviors broken, we are free to seek the misplaced dreams of our youth. There's a quote from Thoreau that states, "Not till we are completely lost, or turned round . . . do we begin to find ourselves . . ."

If Thoreau speaks the truth, then you have begun to play the most elegant and courageous game of "hide-no-more-and-forever-seek" imaginable. You've turned away from hiding the truth, however unpleasant, and have turned instead to life's most rewarding treasure hunt: the search for the best, most constructive, caring, giving, loving person that you can possibly be. You've stepped out of the shadows of conceit and concealment to shine the proverbial light of truth on who you are, what you do, and how you think.

Bravo! It's almost impossible to discuss the changes you've made in plain English. The poetic "warrior of the light" metaphor may be a bit much, but you need to feel your success. So we're going to search long and hard for the exact words to congratulate you on the courage you've displayed in undertaking this life-changing journey.

While there's no merit badge or medal to pin to your chest, the quality of life in the days ahead will be its own reward. Celebrate your commitment to a glorious future by quietly continuing to embrace the beauty in each day. To ensure your forward motion, there is one thing you must do: Stay grateful. Gratitude for all you are given is the fuel that life runs on. Make it a resting place in your busy day. Stop often to acknowledge the gifts you've received.

A deep breath is a rewarding place to start. Close your eyes, breathe deeply, feel your lungs expand with each inhalation, and wonder at your body's ability to convert that oxygen into a substance your blood can carry to all parts of your physical being. *The miracle of our bodies— rejoice.* Say it. *Thank you for this blessed breath. Thank you for this gift.*

When you say these things, you are speaking from the highest place of your mortal being. You become one with this almighty life source as you acknowledge its presence.

Gratitude.

Look around. The spectacular effect of light on surface: color, texture, shape, leaf, tree. Vision. Peripheral vision. Sunlight. Be grateful for the morning as each day comes alive. Sound. Song. Chatter. Traffic. Laughter. Stay grateful for the miracle of hearing. Laughter. Marvel at the way your brain works. How an unexpected action—someone slipping on a banana peel, for example—can be tragic one moment and hilarious the next. Funny. Be grateful for funny. Without funny, we'd all be looking for a ledge.

Gratitude.

Look upon the scars of your broken past as bookmarks to a bit of text you need to remember. It's evidence of a misstep in a direction you won't choose again. A skintight reminder of who you've been and what you've done, and perhaps a measure of how far away from that person you've traveled. Be grateful for having survived. Take the lessons of your fall and the rewards of rising to your full height and share them where you can do the most good. It is your natural instinct to teach what you have learned. We all experience that drive. Honor it wherever you're most needed.

And trust.

You have company. Undefined perhaps. At this point you may be experiencing that warm sense of the invisible companion. Wrap your love around that sensation. Clasp that sense of being cared for in pure love. Feel your love returning to the source of all goodness in a perpetual action as constant as the tide, and find in that bonding of your spirit to that one almighty life source everything you need to live in peace.

Trust.

Believe completely that the unknown will be revealed to you in time if you stay on course and that ultimately you will be led to your own true place. For now, trust that you are exactly where you need to be.

Accept the truth of the moment. Trust the unseen hand on the tiller of your ship. Emmet Fox, the great spiritual leader of the thirties and forties, reminded his listeners that "the captain is on the bridge." It's a lovely thought. Trust that there are eyes that pierce the darkness of your future and that somehow you will be guided to a safe harbor. A *safe harbor*. Such metaphors are inevitable. Warriors of the light are us. It's impossible to avoid such lofty thoughts and dialogue once you've given yourself to this benevolent process—benevolent because in the very seeking of relief we find comfort, and in the sharing of the process we feel enlarged.

The unexamined life has rolled along on autopilot for many of us. Responding again and again from a place of hurt or anger, we seldom took that cleansing breath and examined our intentions before responding. Today the threat of injury, heartache, and self-destructive behavior may be eliminated, or at least diluted by the calming presence of a caring spirit or the touch of invisible hands.

Our actions and reactions are unencumbered by the need to "even the score" or "prove our point," no matter the cost. The quiet mind observes itself and listens for the voice of God. Some things remain too massive to ever understand or explain, but we can imagine. And beyond imagining, we accept that there is simply something wondrous beyond wonder that holds us. We trust that it is there and move forward toward a life that we never imagined. We've learned to give ourselves to a process that remains committed to the highest good of all concerned. There's an anonymous quote that says it beautifully: "Care deeply, give freely, think kindly, act gently, and be at peace with the world."

Gratitude and trust: the birthplace of love.

PAUL'S PERSONAL FREEDOM

Personal freedom. Can you imagine the value I place in those words after decades imprisoned by my addiction? I'm notorious for becoming emotional when speaking of my recovery. Tracey usually sees it coming when I'm about to be touched by some phrase we've written or something she's said about the work we're doing. She'll nod, smile, and announce, "Here comes Weepy Williams." She's usually right.

> "SOMETHING NEEDS TO CHANGE,
> AND IT'S PROBABLY ME."

Two years ago, having slipped into a sedentary lifestyle and being well on my way to fat and unhappy, my son Cole shared his opinion of my condition. "Dad, you're beginning to look like a cookie jar." At 160 pounds and gaining, I was heading for either a heart attack, a stroke, or, at the very least, stretch leisure suits. I remind you that I'm only five foot two. Not who I wanted to be.

Something needed to change. And it was me. I began to monitor and alter my eating habits. I needed to exercise daily. I started running for my life. I dropped thirty pounds, which I've kept off for two years. It worked and continues to work. Something needed to change, and it was me.

We added the *probably* to the first affirmation because in the first investigative moments of change there are sometimes factors that are well outside our control. But there are still many that are ours alone. The *probably* felt honest and even friendlier. Like you could say it and mean it.

When I looked carefully at the how and why of my weight gain, I could find no person or institution to share the blame. It was my own doing. The word *probably* was extraneous. The need for change was all the property of yours truly. If I was going to enjoy the years that remained for me, I would have to change. But the "toe-in-the-water" benefit of that *probably* is undeniable. It allows the process to begin in a softer, gentler way. There is no harsh "guilty-as-charged" self-judgment or sentence of slash and burn. No meat cleaver of "sentenced to a lifetime of favorite food abstinence" slicing into the first few days of redirecting our paths and setting new goals. *Probably* left room for self-examination to begin and willingness to emerge.

Something needs to change, and it's probably me. I said it. I meant it. I began to see results. An expanding waistline was only one of the symptoms of my behavior that would benefit from those words. During the last two years, there has been ample opportunity to employ them. The battle of ego versus humility is an ongoing challenge. Fear emerging as anger or cynicism. The distractions of work or self-interest have sometimes kept me from remaining present as a husband, father, or friend. There have been moments when my actions were unintentionally thoughtless and unkind. Recognizing my poor performance and having an immediate portal to better behavior has been a gift. And always wrapped in gratitude.

> "I DON'T KNOW HOW TO DO THIS
> BUT SOMETHING INSIDE ME DOES."

Years of sobriety and the kindness of other alcoholics were the nourishing soil I trusted to begin a new chapter in my personal transformation. I had another distinct advantage. I had a higher power. I'm a believer. Neil Diamond wrote it; the Monkees made it a part of our lexicon. (An irrelevant side note: I auditioned for the Monkees and was turned down. "No," a gift one more time. I doubt that I'd have enjoyed the career I have if I'd been accepted instead of the talented Davy Jones.)

But, yes, I'm a big believer. I know the comfort and power of trusting in something other than my own visible strengths. In early sobriety, the writings of Emmet Fox were important in my search for divine guidance. Ernest Holmes suggested that "thoughts became things," and that "what we dwell on we create." He also asserted that there is an unseen power that could be tapped into for good or evil. That what we assumed would happen often did because the universe heard our inner belief system as what we desired. "I'll never get that job" was more than just self-doubt. It was a prayer.

"As a man thinketh in his heart, so is he . . ." (Proverbs 23:7). Same deal.

My ability to trust begins with this affirmation. And it swings from the ordinary to the truly mystical—ordinary in the way the unconscious mind works to solve the simplest riddles, like retrieving long-forgotten names and dates, and mystical in ways that are beyond explanation. They're things most of us have experienced but can never fully understand. The thought of a loved one at the exact moment of their passing. The forgotten item that caused you to return to your home only to find the beginnings of a fire. The uneasy feeling about getting on a bus that you hear later crashed.

Each of us will find our own way to truly believing. But the power of intention is at the heart of the second affirmation. I say it often. They play "The Star-Spangled Banner" before ball games; I say the second affirmation before I walk onstage. Or when writing begins with a flourish and grinds to a halt, when a blank piece of paper or computer document feels like a dead end, when the words won't come, I no longer force the issue. I take a little break, look around at the world I'm privileged to live in, take a deep breath, stir in a little gratitude, and speak the truth: "I don't know how to do this but something inside me does."

Again and again, I reaffirm the presence of whatever creative force has given me the words—and sometimes the music—since this journey with Tracey began. For me, my morning run has become my meditation, my entry-level conversation with the Big Amigo. It's where I reiterate *I don't know how to do this but something inside me does.* I've spoken that truth, *knowing* it was an undeniable fact. In my seventies I have seen greater joy, opportunity, and success than I could ever have imagined. It's the glorious impact of trust—complete trust—wrapped in the beauty of gratitude.

> "I WILL LEARN FROM MY MISTAKES
> AND NOT DEFEND THEM."

For me, the third affirmation is a shortcut to responsible adulthood. I was not the quickest to abandon adolescent behavior. The positive results of using this proclamation have made it my favorite. It is also one of the greatest time-savers I've ever employed.

We can't change the past, but I'd love to go back a few decades and holler, "Look, Mom. I'm all grown up. I finally get it." Life can change in that moment when the lights go on, when we truly see that we've screwed up and that it's nobody's fault but our own. It can, and should be, a turning point, a wake-up call.

For many years my mistakes were followed by instant excuses, some invented out of thin air. It's a wheel-spinning task and tap dance that's, frankly, exhausting. It's a nasty little habit many of us share. We keep churning out our most eloquent defenses as time slips away. Sometimes friends do too. And opportunities.

I use this affirmation as quickly and as often as necessary—from rebuilding bridges with friends I've abandoned to repairing online cyber blunders. It's a multipurpose tool that I employ frequently and to great effect. I use this affirmation to lighten my psychic load. Use it to rid myself of a defensive habit that is totally counterproductive. If I'm busy creating believable defenses for my latest errors, I'm not creating art. Or making friends.

> "I WILL MAKE RIGHT THE WRONGS
> I'VE DONE WHEREVER POSSIBLE."

I started doing this work many years ago. It was an essential part of my recovery, my personal freedom. I had to clean up the wreckage of my past if I was ever going to get a good night's sleep.

We've written extensively about the making-amends process. It has been, for me, an action with immediate benefits. I can physically feel my world change when I take that first unburdened breath after fixing something I've broken—the healing energy of putting a relationship shiny side up when my actions left it upside down and ruined.

Some days the world sparkles. It does. When I have admitted my part in some disaster and moved to repair it, I am awestruck by the difference in the way my world shines.

Many times I've found my views of an incident will change with the passing years. A negative event or catastrophe that I had been convinced was never my fault can, when viewed with less ego or passion, suddenly emerge as my responsibility. Facing the facts in a new light, I am reminded by our fourteen-syllable Jiminy Cricket that I need to act. It's never too late to own our mistakes.

> ## "I WILL EXAMINE MY BEHAVIOR
> ## ON A DAILY BASIS."

I've almost always had a regular housecleaning service. I can be a bit of a mess at home, and we need someone to keep things livable. The Fifth Affirmation is the spiritual version of that: a mental maid at the end of the day, slapping at this and that bit of dust that needs cleaning up. It's not the best of metaphors because the work is mine, not someone else's, but you get the idea. It's a gift to be able to end my evening with a long, quiet look at the events of the day and say, "Thank you, Big Amigo. Things are looking shipshape and I am nothing but grateful for that."

And yes, there have been nights in my life when the review of my behavior will pop up a little wart that needs removing. The discipline of regular examination makes the fact that the future is brighter with instant repair the quickest road to peace of mind.

> ## "I WILL LIVE IN LOVE AND SERVICE,
> ## GRATITUDE AND TRUST."

Calling Weepy Williams. The gratitude I feel at this time of my life is monumental. Sharing this task with Tracey has been a gift. Writing this book has truly been a labor of love for us. It began with the phrase *gratitude and trust*. I think I said something to the effect of "My choo-choo runs on twin rails of gratitude and trust" and Tracey responded with "There's a book there." She was right. As usual. And the journey began.

As we created the affirmations, we began to use them. I believe they've made us better people. Really. And they have made life easier. That I know for sure. I have felt the change in myself and seen the change in Tracey.

"I will live my life in love and service." The secret of happiness is in those words. It is for me the easier, softer way. And lest you begin to think of this all as selfless labor, I'll confess something: It's the best, sweetest, and most enjoyable part of being Paul Williams. I have never had more fun. And I have never felt more useful. For years I drank and used to medicate a feeling of being irrelevant. It was an antidote to the fear of feeling "less than" and the feeling of being inches away from being found out as an impostor. An uninvited guest to the party.

I don't know why. I was probably born with it, my "-ism." But the booze and the drugs inflated my ego and allowed me to march on, sleepwalking through my life. Until that glorious day when I woke up. Today I'm wide-awake and running on pure gratitude and trust.

These days I am, for the most part, fearless. Challenges are met with "I don't know how to do this but something inside me does." And after a lifetime of "Look at me," I find the noisy head quiets when I think of helping someone else. The puzzle's easily solved when I turn my attention to some small effort I might make on another's behalf.

Of course, I can be selfish. But I'm less so because I remind myself again and again that the discipline of offering love and service to the world is like ordering dessert—an extra helping of pleasure, peace, and purpose. And, of course, gratitude and trust.

The best of the best has come to me. I am eternally grateful for the life I've lived, and I trust that the future will provide whatever I need to flourish.

What do I do to make this pageantry of safety, peace of mind, joyful opportunity, and meaningful work a constant? I've learned you can't feed tomorrow's hunger with today's food. I must resist the urge to leap into the future and instead return to this perfect now and announce my intentions to the universe.

> "I WILL LIVE IN LOVE AND SERVICE, GRATITUDE AND TRUST."

And so it is. It works. Can I get an amen?

—Paul Williams

TRACEY'S "IN CLOSING"

When Bill W. and Dr. Bob first founded AA, Bill W. said, "Let's keep it simple."

I think that is one of the keys to its success over the decades. When you are looking for a way out, you want a simple road that is clearly marked.

When Paul and I set out to write this book and map out what we felt was the essence of things in the recovery movement that would work for "all people," keeping it simple was foremost on our minds.

Life is complicated enough, and even more so when we are trying to deal with our issues, harness our impulse control, right our wrongs, and figure out where we might have skidded off the rails. Keeping it simple assures us that if we are rigorous in our dedication to change, then we will access these affirmations throughout our days.

I initially said I wanted to write this book because I needed to read it. Over the course of the two years that Paul and I have been working on it, the Six Affirmations of Personal Freedom have become the foundational principles by which I lead my life. I slip up. I am human. But they are so ingrained in me by now, I can find my way back to them even in dark moments. I can and do apply them in situations that have historically pushed all my buttons and sent me catapulting right into formerly comfortable, destructive behavior or caused me to give in to my worst impulses even while declaring I wouldn't.

Habits are automatic responses to either positive or negative stimulation and desires. Once you replace the bad impulses with the good ones, you will find yourself going there first, time and time again.

> "SOMETHING NEEDS
> TO CHANGE."

I have a tendency to be impatient. I wouldn't say I get angry easily. I'm not physical or abusive. I get frustrated. I get irritated. I get anxious that things are not going according to my plan. That plan can be as minor as printing up my day's work to as big a deal as a doctor overlooking something serious and endangering my health.

I have a lifelong tendency to get exasperated when dealing with anyone who I think is not doing their job well, pulling their weight, acting responsibly, or playing by my rules. I think *my rules* are the defining words in that statement. I have had an "It's my way or the highway" attitude for much of my life.

I used to be in a pretty continuous state of agitation, as most people tend not to do things exactly the way you want. I then felt a profound need to tell off whoever was dishing out the incompetence. I seldom gave others the benefit of thought; I gave a piece of my mind instead.

This has done me far more harm than good. I have angered flight attendants, teachers, people I've worked with . . . the list goes on. You could say there was even a dose of "When I got to the fork in the road, I took the knife" in my responses at times.

I can be quick-tongued, and I have been lightning-fast when it came to pressing the SEND button or telling someone what they did wrong, how they needed to do it right, and how their actions not only disrupted my world order but often sent the entire planet off its axis.

This was entirely my fault. Well, easy there, girl, maybe not my fault—as people do act like nincompoops much of the time. But I am not the chief of police for the planet. And what may seem nincompoopish to me might be someone else operating at their highest level. What was my fault was the way I dealt with it.

> "I WILL LEARN FROM MY MISTAKES
> AND NOT DEFEND THEM."

Would it hurt the people who work at airports to tell you how late the plane is going to be when they do, in fact, know, as opposed to staring at you and saying, "We will let you know closer to the time of departure"? Boy, have I blown up at them. In fact, my family used to bet on how long it would take me to tell off the guy at Jet Blue who was not running things the way I would.

Authority figures are my bête noire, and I know exactly where it comes from—straight from my childhood, straight from feeling helpless in the face of my father and his dismissal. I felt helpless in not being able to say what I thought or felt and have it be heard or given the space it needed.

But a big part of this work is moving forward and not blaming the present on the past. It is not okay for me to yell at the people at the cable company because the cable is out and they don't know when it will be fixed. It is not okay for me to walk around holding on to anger from my past and using it as a hand grenade on others in my present.

We make peace with our past by facing it, accepting it, and moving on accordingly. We can identify the triggers, but we cannot use them as our excuses for whatever we are doing that is not right. "Something needs to change, and it's probably me" is probably the step I go to most frequently. If it's my attitude, my take on the situation, my need for control, my desire to have it go my way, or my inability to see it from the other person's side, I immediately stop and repeat that affirmation. I then look at how I can change myself within the situation.

In the two years I have been using these affirmations, there have been hundreds of examples where I stop myself and say, "Something needs to change, and it's probably me." It took me a while to make it the first action I take in an uncomfortable state. I might have declared it, but old habits take time to modify. This is a one-day-at-a-time process. And there were occasions where I might have said, "I was the one that needed to change," but my behavior did not follow suit. And in those times I would find myself having to leapfrog my way directly to "I will make right the wrongs wherever possible." I would have to make amends for whatever my part was.

> ### "I WILL MAKE RIGHT THE WRONGS I'VE DONE WHEREVER POSSIBLE"

I found this shortcut an excuse for a bad attitude. Let's say I was chewing out the guy on the other end of the phone at Time Warner Cable. I would preface my tirade with "I know this is not your fault, you only work there, but I'm mad as hell and this is why." It's kind of a feeble way to justify poor behavior, but it's better than looking like you're mean and unexamined. *But you know, if I lose it, I apologize in that minute.* We all know when we are back in the gray zone, and we understand that we have to rectify it as quickly as possible. Saves a lot of time, a lot of hurt feelings, and a lot of beating ourselves up—or, worse yet, making excuses for why behaved the way we did.

Something needs to change, and it's probably me. By training myself to say it often, it eventually became my go-to mantra. When I feel upset, disoriented, wronged, or hurt; when things are not going the way I want; when I find myself up against a wall, and an old uncomfortable response or emotion is on the tip of my tongue or beating in my heart, I go to "Something needs to change, and it's probably me."

I use it in the bigger relationships in my life as well as the daily annoyances. I have had to employ it with my oldest child. She is growing up. It's hard to let her go. I was pulling and she was pushing. Something needed to change, and it was my grasp on her. Once I did that, she came bouncing back. It's the first thing I say to myself when my world starts to slide a bit sideways.

The funny thing is, for a control freak, it is actually the perfect position to take, as the only thing any of us has any control over is our own behavior. So by going right to the stance of *Something needs to change, and it's probably me*, we rip that power right back to our side. It sounds like tossing in the towel, but it's the reverse. It is the most commanding rock we can plant ourselves on.

I can be paranoid too. As I said, I am programmed to reach for a bottle of disappointment. If I don't hear back from someone right away, I immediately think, *I must have upset them. They are mad at me. I did something wrong. Now they might disappear.* That distrust takes me to the familiar place of being abandoned: *Wait, I can't let that happen, so I will be the dumper as opposed to the dumpee. Who needs them anyway?* Then I laundry list all the reasons why I don't really want them in my life. When I find myself going to that place now, I stop. I look at the situation. I say to myself, *Something needs to change, and it's probably me.* Sometimes that will immediately lead me to pondering what the other person's side might be. Since we do live in the center of our own universe, it is not always easy to try and imagine what is going on with someone else. If we are prone to suspicion and mistrust, our knee-jerk reaction is to react—from the fear, not from the truth of the moment. But the affirmations allow you to stop before action. If used consistently and properly, the affirmations are a hedge between you and your impulses. Your impulse to yell, write someone off, spend too much money, have that drink, have that extra burger, press SEND without thinking of the ramifications, take it out on your kids, your dog, your mate, yourself. They allow you to stop and access everything from a place of clarity and not old, worn-out emotions.

What part of this is my stuff? Often, most of it. Even if it's just your reaction.

Sometimes, like many of us, I go to a dark, familiar cubbyhole of pain and self-pity or the *Oh, the world is not being nice to Tracey* place. From that height or depth, it's harder to instantly change me. That's when I go to *I don't know how to do this but something inside me does.* That calms me. It allows me to drift to a less choppy shore and just be, just trust.

> "I DON'T KNOW HOW TO DO THIS BUT SOMETHING INSIDE ME DOES."

My spiritual life has always tilted a bit toward *God is everywhere,* so sticking that trust in my core assures me I am never without it. And it really does allow me to just let go. Just go with it. Stop kicking, screaming, wanting, pushing and demanding. Just live quietly in trust. Wait for a sign. Know it's okay sometimes to do nothing, to let someone/ something else take over.

Sometimes it's enough to just stop and breathe. Other times I might walk into a church, any church, and feel the presence of so many hearts beating the drum of belief. There's a large church steeple outside my office window, and sometimes I will sit back and stare at it. And know there is something out there that is bigger than me, than my will, than my past, than my fears or what I think will make me happy in the moment, and I let it go. Letting it go. Handing it over. Just being. One of life's great lessons, though easier to proclaim than to follow through on. But again, when you continue to do it, it becomes the way you think, the way you respond. You go there. You know how to get to faith the same way you know how to get yourself home. And faith then becomes your address.

If you asked me my favorite affirmation outside of gratitude and trust, it is without a doubt

> **"I WILL MAKE RIGHT THE WRONGS I'VE DONE WHEREVER POSSIBLE."**

Hello, clean slate. Bye-bye, guilt. Enter the world of being a responsible adult and good riddance to the petulant child who thinks it's everyone's fault but her own. Accountability rules!

I just love this. I love doing it. I love being on the receiving end of it. I know for a fact there was a time in my life when I had hoped, wished—dreamed—that people would apologize to me for hurts they caused. I have let that go. But I do remember the feeling. I also recall what is felt like to carry the weight of my misdeeds, to want to say sorry. And I know how envious I was of my friend Blake when he roamed through all the back rooms of his life making right all his wrongs. I recall how peaceful he felt, how burden-free. When you are a person of conscience, as most people are, you know where you have screwed up.

We can name the people we have wounded. We carry that around. It is such a relief to rid yourself of that burden and move forward light of step and open of heart.

I will learn from my mistakes and not defend them and *I will examine my behavior on a daily basis* are the affirmations that helped me curb my shopping habit. I needed to put the brakes on. I sat down and looked at all my charges for a year. It was hard. You know those year-end statements? I would hide them. I would. I did not want to face that music. But one day I just opened them and looked at them. I circled all the things I knew were superfluous impulse purchases, things that were already in the bag for Goodwill. Things I didn't need or could not justify; things that simply fed the beast of addiction. And I listed them.

I then took six months and paid off all my charges. I made one bank account for my shopping money. No mingling, no charging one thing on this card, one thing on another. At the beginning of the month, that account gets a certain amount, some months more than others, depending on family expenses. Sometimes I take a side job of script analyzing and that goes in there. That is my shopping allowance. And I did the thing they tell you to do: I cut up most of my cards.

I committed myself to the process.

And the great thing is, now I enjoy shopping more. I enjoy my purchases more. They are not impulsive or random, and they are not material excuses for something I think I am missing. They are deliberate and accounted for. And I am accountable for them. It's a great feeling.

Oh, gratitude and trust—either one alone is nourishment for the soul. Together they are the dynamic duo that, when incorporated into your daily life, have the ability to turn any situation into a blessing. I know that is a hard one to believe. Maybe not for the real believers, but for the doubters, it is a big dive into the unknown waters of the devotion pool—but it does work.

> "I WILL LIVE IN LOVE AND SERVICE,
> GRATITUDE AND TRUST."

Just look at the people who live their lives in love and service. They need little else. They do not worry, they do not fret, they don't feel a lack. When you trust, you eliminate fear and find yourself living in the moment. If you are living in the moment, you can focus on joy and gratitude. Once you land on gratitude, it's all a gift. With gratitude, you feel compelled to share it.

I used to be very hung up on who I was and how the world perceived me. When I was a screenwriter, I was very externally focused and always worrying about the day it would all disappear. And, of course, one day it did. As things do. I found myself having to reinvent myself in midlife. I was devastated for a spell. What would I do? Who was I if I wasn't a screenwriter? What would I tell people? How would it look? I made people laugh. Now what would I do?

I was always working toward some end. My life was made up of "If this happened, then maybe that would happen"—it was a lot of two ifs and many maybes. It was always life in the future lane. I lived for what might happen down the line. That is what the movie business is all about.

Now I wake up and every day I live my life in love and service. If ten years ago anyone had told me that I would end up here, doing this, I would have said they were nuts. Yes, sometimes my ego jumps on the stage. I have one. It's not that well hidden. But when it happens, I quickly remind myself I live my life in gratitude and trust and love and service. And the reassertion of those principles is all that I need to put me back on course. As Paul wrote in the song for *Bugsy Malone*, "You give a little love and it all comes back to you." That pretty much sums it up.

Stay strong. Stay focused. Live in the moment. Do not give in to your worst impulses. Make right your wrongs. Live responsibly and with faith. Give a little love to yourself and those you come in contact with, and you will be amazed at the quality of your life.

Blessings,

—*Tracey Jackson*

Acknowledgments

This book, like most every decent idea I come up with, started in the shower. I am eternally grateful for the aquatic chamber that allows my mind to slow down and ideas to take flight.

But ideas remain only ideas without the effort, imagination, and faith of many people.

I have to start with thanking my writing partner for taking this on and not thinking I was crazy when I proposed it. Paul had to take some big steps of bravery to sign on to this book. And the collaboration has been a highlight of my working life.

Most books would remain desktop files if not for the support of a good agent. Eric Simonoff is the best. I'm grateful you are my agent, and the mere mention of your name instantly bumps up my author status.

All publishers are not created equal, and David Rosenthal is one of a kind. He is as tough as he is kind. He is fair and he protects the integrity of the project. He "got" this book in ways we never did. Because David thinks out of the box, he allows his writers to do the same and I remain eternally grateful.

"Team Blue Rider" brought this book into the world, Sarah Hochman, Phoebe Pickering, Aileen Boyle, Eliza Rosenberry, thank you for your wisdom, assistance, encouragement, and hard work: And an extra spoonful of gratitude for responding to my late-night e-mails and endless requests. Jason Booher, a round of applause and gratitude for designing the perfect book jacket on the first try.

Rachel Holtzman worked diligently by my side to edit this book. She is living proof that multitasking can work as she edited the book, took care of her baby, and moved to Chicago all in the same week. Thank you for being open, wise, and faster than the speed of light. You need a cape with SE for Super Editor on it.

Sandi Mendolson, I could not do many of the things I do without you. Well, I could do them, but nobody would ever know I had.

And there is always the chorus standing behind you. Michele Rowe for opening yourself up in a time of great turmoil and for always being such a cheerleader. My cousin, AJ Jacobs, for believing in this project from its infancy and through its terrible twos.

Steppie, John Henry, Irwin, and all our wonderful followers at gratitudeandtrust.com; you have been a loving, engaged group of teachers. You thought we were teaching you things, but you were informing us of what people needed to hear and how they needed to hear it. You have been and remain invaluable to our mission.

And then, always last in these things, but never least, my family, Glenn, Taylor, and Lucy, and my mother, Beverley, who love me in spite of who I am. Help to be the best self I can be. Forgive me when I falter and are an endless source of material. I love you all for more than you will ever understand.

—Tracey Jackson

This book, and any good that comes from its publication, is the direct result of my partnership with a tireless, inspired, relentless, sometimes impossible woman named Tracey Jackson. It is the child of her devotion to getting it done and getting it done right.

It was her idea to write it. Sparked by my use of the words "gratitude and trust" she suggested we team tackle this wonderful task together. I'm grateful for the chance to take this, my first literary journey, with such a remarkable friend.

I'm also grateful for her willingness to go to any lengths to respect and protect my relationship to the sacred world of recovery. Sincere thanks to Penguin Blue Rider for doing the same. There are remarkable and generous men, women, and organizations who'd rather not have their names printed for the world to see. Many of the people most deserving of my acknowledged gratitude will remain anonymous.

But there are others who've seasoned my life with beautiful ideas. Their wisdom lives on in my language and my actions. Dr. Jim Turrell, my friend and minister at the Center for Spiritual Living, is an inspired coach and guide. That "something inside me knows" affirmation is solidly attached to his teaching. He's made me feel capable of things that seemed impossible. It's why I continue to golf.

The many names that Tracey mentioned need to be read aloud with reverence and respect here too. Our publisher, David Rosenthal, felt like a trusted friend from the very beginning. When Tracey and I decided to write in a combined singular voice, David suggested the individual boxes that would allow us to tell our own stories and the life lessons they contained. A man of solutions and insight.

Thanks to Sarah Hochman, Phoebe Pickering, Aileen Boyle, and Eliza Rosenberry for their expertise, and, of course, Jason Booher for the lean and meaningful design.

Rachel Holtzman worked closely with Tracey to complete the task of editing and preparing the book for publication. It was heavy lifting, labor intensive, and I was of little or no help. I'm grateful that the work was accomplished so skillfully under difficult personal conditions.

Eric Simonoff, Tracey's agent, welcomed me into his literary stable. Thank you, sir. You took up the task of representing a newbie with ease and grace.

The men and women who've become part of the Gratitude and Trust family at www.gratitudeandtrust.com have given us support and valuable feedback. Thanks to all of you.

I'm nominating Glenn Horowitz and Mariana Williams for sainthood. They've displayed superhuman amounts of patience, flexibility, and willingness to endure opposing inconveniences. I spent weeks at a time in New York working with Tracey. Mariana faced an empty chair at the dinner table while Tracey's husband, Glenn, graciously accepted an extra setting at his.

Glenn, Taylor, and Lucy made me feel like a member of the family and I will always be grateful.

Mariana, you remained loving, tolerant, and always supportive of what you said would be my "legacy of love" for recovery. You saw this work as meaningful and important. I love you for seeing its potential. Thanks to you, Darin and Julia too.

Thanks to my brother Mentor for always living up to his name.

My greatest source of pride will always be my daughter Sarah and son Cole. I've joked that you did a great job of raising me. You live in my heart. I could write a book about how proud I am of you.

To my associates at ASCAP, especially John LoFrumento and Nancy Munoz, thank you for your support and assistance in keeping me shiny side up during some crazy times.

Finally, thank you to the choir of grateful hearts that came before, welcomed me into their healing circle, and showed me a new way of living. To the recovering alcoholics and addicts who loved me back to life I send blessings and thanks. I'll keep coming back.

—*Paul Williams*